Helping Kids in Crisis

Managing Psychiatric Emergencies in Children and Adolescents

Helping Kids in Crisis

Managing Psychiatric Emergencies in Children and Adolescents

Edited by

Fadi Haddad, M.D.
Ruth Gerson, M.D.

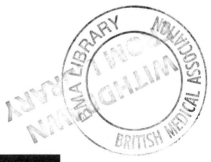

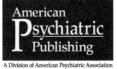

American
Psychiatric
Publishing
A Division of American Psychiatric Association

Washington, DC
London, England

If you would like to buy between 25 and 99 copies of this or any other American Psychiatric Publishing title, you are eligible for a 20% discount; please contact Customer Service at appi@psych.org or 800-368-5777. If you wish to buy 100 or more copies of the same title, please e-mail us at bulksales@psych.org for a price quote.

Copyright © 2015 American Psychiatric Association
ALL RIGHTS RESERVED

Manufactured in the United States of America on acid-free paper
18 17 16 15 14   5 4 3 2 1
First Edition

Typeset in Adobe's Baskerville BE and Formatta

American Psychiatric Publishing
A Division of American Psychiatric Association
1000 Wilson Boulevard
Arlington, VA 22209-3901
www.appi.org

Library of Congress Cataloging-in-Publication Data
Helping kids in crisis (Haddad)
   Helping kids in crisis : managing psychiatric emergencies in children and adolescents / edited by Fadi Haddad, Ruth S. Gerson. – First edition.
      p. ; cm.
   Includes bibliographical references and index.
   ISBN 978-1-58562-482-9 (pbk. : alk. paper)
   I. Haddad, Fadi, editor. II. Gerson, Ruth, editor.
III. American Psychiatric Association, issuing body. IV. Title.
[DNLM: 1. Emergency Services, Psychiatric. 2. Mental Disorders–therapy.
3. Adolescent. 4. Child. 5. Crisis Intervention. WS 350.2]
   RC480.6
   616.89'025–dc23   2014030047

British Library Cataloguing in Publication Data
A CIP record is available from the British Library.

To the children and families who have taught us
so much along the way

Contents

Contributors

Maggie Bielsky, LMSW
Inpatient Psychiatric Social Worker, Department of Child and Adolescent Psychiatry, Bellevue Hospital Center, New York, New York

Gabrielle S. Carson, Ph.D.
Clinical Psychologist and Clinical Instructor, NYU School of Medicine, Department of Child and Adolescent Psychiatry, Bellevue Hospital Children's Comprehensive Psychiatric Emergency Program, New York, New York

Ruth Gerson, M.D.
Director, Bellevue Hospital Children's Comprehensive Psychiatric Emergency Program; Clinical Assistant Professor, Department of Child and Adolescent Psychiatry, NYU School of Medicine, New York, New York

Charles J. Glawe, M.D.
Clinical Assistant Professor of Child and Adolescent Psychiatry, NYU School of Medicine; Unit Chief, Bellevue Hospital Adolescent Inpatient Service, New York, New York

Fadi Haddad, M.D.
Director Emeritus, Bellevue Hospital Children's Comprehensive Psychiatric Emergency Program; Clinical Assistant Professor, Department of Child and Adolescent Psychiatry, NYU School of Medicine, New York, New York

Jennifer F. Havens, M.D.
Vice Chair for Public Psychiatry, Department of Child and Adolescent Psychiatry, NYU School of Medicine; Director and Chief of Service, Department of Child and Adolescent Psychiatry, Bellevue Hospital Center, New York, New York

Alessandra D.E. Herbosch, Psy.D.
Clinical and Forensic Psychologist, Bellevue Hospital, New York, New York

Rachel Mandel, M.D.
Assistant Clinical Professor, Department of Child and Adolescent Psychiatry, NYU School of Medicine; Attending Psychiatrist, Bellevue Hospital Children's Comprehensive Psychiatric Emergency Program, New York, New York

Mollie C. Marr, B.F.A.
Program Coordinator, Bellevue Innovation Lab, Department of Child and Adolescent Psychiatry, NYU School of Medicine, Bellevue Hospital Center, New York, New York

Jasmine Marrero, LCSW
Psychiatric Social Work Supervisor, Children's Comprehensive Psychiatric Emergency Program, Department of Child and Adolescent Psychiatry, Bellevue Hospital Center, New York, New York

Melissa Negron, LCSW
Psychiatric Social Worker, Children's Comprehensive Psychiatric Emergency Program, Department of Child and Adolescent Psychiatry, Bellevue Hospital Center, New York, New York

Stephen Ross, M.D.
Director, Division of Alcoholism and Drug Abuse, Bellevue Hospital Center; Director, Addiction Psychiatry, NYU Tisch Hospital; Department of Psychiatry, Bellevue Hospital Center, NYU Langone Medical Center, New York, New York

Susan B. Torrey, M.D.
Director, Division of Pediatric Emergency Medicine, Department of Emergency Medicine; Associate Professor of Emergency Medicine and Pediatrics (Clinical), NYU School of Medicine, New York, New York

M. Cevdet Tosyali, M.D.
Director, Adolescent Psychiatry Inpatient Service, Department of Child and Adolescent Psychiatry, Bellevue Hospital Center; Clinical Assistant Professor, Department of Child and Adolescent Psychiatry, NYU School of Medicine, New York, New York

J. Rebecca Weis, M.D.
Clinical Assistant Professor, Department of Child and Adolescent Psychiatry, NYU School of Medicine; Director of Early Childhood Mental Health Service, Bellevue Hospital Center, New York, New York

Introduction

Children who are experiencing behavioral crises have often had escalating symptoms that overwhelm and frighten them, and their families have exhausted their usual support and coping mechanisms. These situations may reach desperate proportions in diverse venues. A child in the classroom may assault another student. One of your patients may disclose suicidal thoughts to you during a routine visit. As the professionals who are providing services to these children, we must be able to quickly determine threats to safety and initiate interventions to de-escalate behaviors, often with limited resources.

Reports from the National Institute of Mental Health and the World Health Organization (WHO) indicate that the number of children with mental health diagnoses is increasing worldwide, with WHO estimating that neuropsychiatric disorders will be one of the top five causes of pediatric morbidity, mortality, and disability by 2020. Similarly, primary care providers have identified a significant increase in the number of psychosocial problems diagnosed in their practices. At the same time, there has been a steady decline in the availability of psychiatric services, both inpatient and outpatient, for children and adults. As a result, more and more children in behavioral crisis are referred to emergency departments, where processes and facilities may be limited, creating a suboptimal environment for their care. Although the majority of children will be discharged home, they typically must wait for prolonged periods in disruptive environments that may escalate their symptoms (Dolan and Fein 2011).

The vast majority of children with psychiatric conditions who reach an emergency department are diagnosed with either aggressive behavior or suicidal ideation. In a large, multicenter retrospective study (Mahajan et al. 2009), 80% of children who came to the emergency departments with psychiatric diagnoses were 10 years or older. Their diagnoses varied by age, with conduct disturbances predominating in those children under 10 years and depressive and neurotic conditions more prevalent among older children. A small but significant number of children 5 years and older had conditions with psychotic features. The admission rate for children in this study was 30%.

These data suggest that most children who are experiencing behavioral crises will not need inpatient treatment. However, practitioners in school or outpatient medical environments are often even more challenged than emergency departments to manage these situations. Facilities resources may be limited. Where can you physically isolate an aggressive child? There may not be processes in place to delineate a graded response for escalating behaviors. Staff may feel unprepared to assess behavioral and environmental risks. In addition, diagnosis-based approaches are not practical in settings where children with different diagnoses are exhibiting similar behaviors and staff may not be mental health professionals.

Helping Kids in Crisis: Managing Psychiatric Emergencies in Children and Adolescents is a practical, symptom-based guide. It will be useful to practitioners in hospital or community-based settings, including physicians in training, pediatricians who work in office-based or emergency settings, psychologists, social workers, school psychologists, guidance counselors, and school nurses. The first portion of the book focuses on clinical care. The initial chapter is devoted to assessing safety and identifying children who should be referred to the emergency department. Subsequent chapters are designed to provide clinical information as well as a practical approach for risk assessment, onsite stabilization, and when to get help. In many of the chapters, these practical suggestions are summarized in easy-to-use algorithms. The book concludes with a discussion of systems issues such as identifying resources for children and families and models of emergency psychiatric care for children.

The Children's Comprehensive Psychiatric Emergency Program at Bellevue Hospital Center is a regional referral center for children with psychiatric emergencies. The editors and authors have practiced in this setting for many years. With the publication of *Helping Kids in Crisis,* those of us on the frontlines can take advantage of their expertise and experience to more effectively and compassionately care for this challenging population.

Susan B. Torrey, M.D.

References

Dolan ME, Fein JA; Committee on Pediatric Emergency Medicine: Pediatric and adolescent mental health emergencies in the emergency medical services system. Pediatrics 127(5):e1356–e1366, 2011

Mahajan P, Alpern ER, Grupp-Phelan J, et al: Epidemiology of psychiatric-related visits to emergency departments in a multicenter collaborative research pediatric network. Pediatr Emergency Care 25(11):715–720, 2009

Acknowledgments

We would like to thank our families and colleagues for their support. We would also like to thank Donna Somma, Esq., for her help in making this book possible.

Disclosure of Conflicting Interests

The following contributors to this book have indicated a financial interest in or other affiliation with a commercial supporter, a manufacturer of a commercial product, a provider of a commercial service, a nongovernmental organization, and /or a government agency, as listed below:

Stephen Ross, M.D.—*Research funding:* Heffter Research Institute, National Institute on Drug Abuse; *Unpaid board member:* Heffter Research Institute.

The following contributors to this book have indicated no competing interests to disclose during the year preceding manuscript submission:

Maggie Bielsky, LMSW
Gabrielle S. Carson, Ph.D.
Ruth Gerson, M.D.
Charles J. Glawe, M.D.
Fadi Haddad, M.D.
Alessandra D. E. Herbosch, Psy.D.
Rachel Mandel, M.D.
Jasmine Marrero, LCSW
Melissa Negron, LCSW
Susan B. Torrey, M.D.
M. Cevdet Tosyali, M.D.
J. Rebecca Weis, M.D.

CHAPTER 1

Kids in Crisis

Fadi Haddad, M.D.

Mental and emotional well-being among children and youths is essential to a productive and meaningful life. Positive mental health strengthens a young person's ability to have healthy relationships, promotes adaptive decision making, and makes the individual resilient and better able to cope with the challenges or adversities of life.

Unfortunately, while we like to think of childhood as a happy and stress-free time, it is a period of significant vulnerability to mental health problems that can disrupt critical aspects of biological, psychological, and social development. According to the Centers for Disease Control and Prevention, 13%–20% of children living in the United States experience a mental disorder in a given year (Perou et al. 2013). Such mental health problems have broad effects on a child's life if left untreated, including problems at home in the child's overall functioning and in relationships with parents and siblings, truancy and academic failures, aggressive or self-harming behaviors, and social difficulties, including isolation and vulnerability to unhealthy relationships. Effective mental health treatment, particularly if given early in the child's illness, can get the child back on track and prevent future mental health problems.

But children and adolescents who are struggling with mental health problems, and their families, often have difficulty accessing the help they need. In many areas of the country, appropriate psychiatric treatment is not available, or the clinics that provide such treatment have long wait lists (Thomas 2003) or high copays, or only take certain types of insurance. Even

1

when services are available, the child and his or her family may not recognize that the child is experiencing a mental illness, may not know how to get treatment, or may be reluctant to seek help because of the stigma that surrounds mental illness. Thus, for many children, mental health problems go unrecognized or untreated until there is a crisis that lands these children in an emergency room (ER). Although obviously children in crisis need treatment, a crisis is the worst time to start mental health treatment—both the child and the family are in acute distress, necessary information from school or pediatricians may not be available, and the child and family may be asked to make difficult decisions with little time to think or process what is happening.

The ER is also often a bad place to start psychiatric treatment. The ER can be scary and stressful. The influx of children in psychiatric crisis, in addition to children seeking medical attention, makes the ER crowded, so that families often have to wait for a long time (Pittsenbarger and Mannix 2014). In most parts of the country, psychiatric evaluation of children is done in the medical or pediatric ER or in the adult psychiatric ER. Both can be frightening for children—there may be acutely medically ill children, or agitated or psychotic adults, in the beds nearby—and often the staff who are there are not trained in working with kids or with mental health problems. The ER staff may have little time to spend with patients and families. The ER has to be efficient during triage in determining which patients are the most acutely and severely ill and devoting attention and resources to those patients. Often psychiatric evaluation in the ER consists of a quick decision to admit (to an inpatient psychiatric unit or to a pediatrics unit if a psychiatric bed is not available) or discharge (ideally, but not always, with a referral for outpatient care). In the best-case scenario, the ER staff will try to collect information from the parents, school, outpatient mental health providers, and others involved with the child to make a thorough assessment and determine the best treatment plan, but sometimes those individuals are not available and the ER has to make a quick decision.

The goal of this volume is to assist those who work with children—teachers, guidance counselors, pediatricians, social workers, community mental health providers, and others—to recognize the early warning signs of impending mental health crisis and help kids get help so that the crisis (and the trip to the ER) can be averted. It will also provide tools for managing a crisis, learning from it, making the most of an ER visit if it is truly needed, and preventing future incidents to help kids stay safe and stay on track.

What Is a Psychiatric Crisis?

Some crises are easy to spot–when a child has tried to kill himself, for example. But in general it is easier to define a medical emergency than a psychiatric one. Although in most cases of medical emergencies the need for seeking immediate help is clear to the individual and the caregivers around him or her, psychiatric symptoms–even acute ones–can be more subtle and internal, or can be misunderstood as "attention-seeking," normal adolescent misbehavior, drug use, or other factors. A psychiatric crisis can come on gradually, with problem behaviors or symptoms escalating over time, making it harder to see when things have reached a crisis point, or it can seemingly come out of nowhere or be evident only at home or only at school.

Agreeing on when to seek mental health evaluation and treatment for a child can be challenging (Janssens et al. 2013). There are huge variations in behavioral norms based on age, developmental milestones, language ability, and parenting and school styles that could make the decision to seek mental health assessment and treatment very difficult. Parents or teachers may disagree about the child's behaviors and symptoms, whether they are severe, what the source of the behavior is, and what the solution should be. In certain situations, it is clear that there is an immediate need for help, such as in the case of a suicide attempt or a severe aggressive outburst at school. But even in such situations, we find differences in opinions, especially between parents and teachers, about the need for sending the child to an ER. At times it is very difficult for a parent to realize that his or her child might need mental health treatment. Sometimes there are two parents who disagree about what their child needs. At other times, the parents are clear that their child needs mental health treatment, but they do not want to be seen in an ER or do not want the child to take medication, or they do want their child to receive medication but do not want him or her to receive necessary educational interventions or social services. For other kids, the parents and school staff may be in agreement, but outpatient providers (pediatricians, therapists, or psychiatrists), family services workers, law enforcement, or others may be recommending a different treatment plan. Unfortunately, kids often get caught in the middle of such disagreements, and treatment is delayed until the situation becomes acute and forces a crisis.

In other cases, the child himself or herself may be the sticking point. While teenagers occasionally do walk into the ER asking for help on their own, this is rare, and often it takes all of the adults in a child's life coming together to support the child for the child to feel safe opening up about his or her difficulties and accepting care. If this does not happen, the child's symptoms are likely to continue to worsen until the child ends up in the ER.

As psychiatric ER providers, we see patients with a wide range of symptoms being referred to the ER for evaluation and intervention (Levine and Najara 2010). Usually these children are referred by schools, parents, foster care agencies, departments of family services, outpatient providers (pediatricians, therapists, psychiatrists), family court, law enforcement, or group homes. The reasons for the referrals vary and can include

- Verbal or physical aggression toward others at school, in a therapist's office, or at home with parents and siblings
- Threats of aggression at school, even without any actual aggressive or agitated behaviors
- Suicidal statements voiced to a parent or teacher, posted on social media, texted to a friend, or written in a journal
- Self-injurious behaviors such as cutting or burning
- Reports of hearing voices or seeing things that are not there
- Tantrums or severe oppositionality at school
- Odd behaviors such as illogical or bizarre behavior, repetitive or compulsive behaviors, or strange ways of interacting socially, such as those seen in autism spectrum disorder
- Severe depression or anxiety
- Risky behaviors such as running away from home or school or risky sexual behaviors
- Drug use (or concern that a change in thinking or behavior may be due to drug use, intoxication, or withdrawal)
- Violence or gang involvement
- Concern for child abuse or other trauma
- Law enforcement involvement, related either to criminal behavior, truancy, running away, or bizarre behavior in a public place or to mandated treatment directed by family court

All of these reasons for referral qualify to be defined as crisis. The thresholds for the referrals depend on the severity of the symptoms and the experience level and comfort zone of the outpatient professional or the referring agency.

When Is a Psychiatric Crisis an Emergency?

Not every crisis qualifies as a psychiatric emergency. Luckily, true psychiatric emergencies are few in number; they involve situations in which there is imminent danger to self or others, such as suicidal or homicidal thoughts with intent and plan, acutely dangerous behaviors that cannot be contained outside of the hospital, or a severe break with reality such that the individual cannot safely navigate the world outside the hospital. Most psychiatric crises are not truly emergencies, and with close coordination among school staff, parents, and others working with the child to give the right interventions and supports early on, the crisis can be managed outside the hospital without a trip to the ER. Sometimes a psychiatric crisis is severe enough that it is clearly an emergency, and a risk assessment in the ER is warranted. This volume will help you as outpatient mental health care providers and other professionals identify ways to manage different types of psychiatric crises and to know when a trip to the ER is really needed.

Expectations From the Emergency Room

When a patient is sent to the ER, the referring agency or professional usually has certain expectations. Generally, the hope is that the child will be kept in the hospital either for a few days of observation or for a few weeks of inpatient hospitalization, and then be connected with intensive outpatient services that will begin immediately on discharge. Unfortunately, these expectations are not in line with what hospitals can actually provide. Most children who are evaluated in the ER for psychiatric emergencies are discharged that same day. Sometimes outpatient referrals will be made, but some ERs do not have the staff or the expertise to make such referrals. In other cases, a child will be held for 24 hours but then discharged if there is not an inpatient bed available, if insurance does not approve a hospitalization, or if the child's condition does not fully meet criteria for an inpatient hospitalization (the criteria being children with severe mental illness who are unable to manage in the community or children who are acutely and imminently dangerous to self or others). In these cases hospital staff will generally try to make referrals for outpatient treatment, but it is rare that such services are immediately available because of wait lists and issues of insurance coverage.

When the patient is discharged from the ER in this way, the referring professional or the family might sense that they were not heard and that their concerns or complaints were dismissed and not addressed properly. Unfortunately, it is very common that a school or outpatient therapist feels a child needs a "higher level of care," but that criteria for an inpatient hospitalization are still not met or inpatient hospitalization is not available in that community or with the child's insurance. At other times, the ER staff are in agreement about a child's need for treatment but the parents disagree and want the child managed as an outpatient or even discharged without any psychiatric follow-up. Managing the different expectations is not an easy mission. The ER staff has to deal with these differing expectations and the conflicts that result and strive to provide the maximum help for the individual and the family within the constraints identified above.

Understanding the Emergency Room Evaluation

While the ER is unlikely to meet all the expectations of those who send a child for evaluation, there may be ways that families, schools, and others who work with kids can work more effectively with ER staff to get the most out of an ER evaluation. Understanding what types of evaluation the ER will do and what information ER staff need will make the family a more effective partner in this process and will help you to ensure that the child gets the help he or she needs.

The ER staff have to be very efficient in their evaluation because of the small window for getting the job done. The patient in the ER is evaluated for a few hours before a decision has to be made, which as noted earlier is generally to admit the child to the hospital, discharge him or her to the community with outside referrals, or keep the child for further observation in the ER. To get the evaluation done in the most efficient way, teamwork is crucial. The clinical staff in the ER have to function differently than other mental health professionals because of limitations of time, overcrowding in the ER, and often the lack of necessary information from schools or providers outside the hospital after-hours. It is not unusual for a school or foster care agency to send a student to the ER for an evaluation, accompanied by a staff person who does not know the details of the incident or any other information about the patient. If the evaluation time happens to be after school or business hours, it may be impossible to get any further information about the details of the incident or the child. This information could be critical in determining if the child should stay in the hospital or could leave with recommendation for outpatient treatment. Conducting the evaluation with missing information is like trying to solve a jigsaw puzzle with missing pieces.

To make a full evaluation, the ER staff have to assess and understand a number of factors in the child's medical, social, and psychiatric history. These include

- Reason for the referral
- Chronological history and the nature of the symptoms
- Any and all stressors at home, at school, in relationships, and so forth

- History of past symptoms, diagnosis, treatments, and medications
- Family psychiatric and social history
- Developmental history, including developmental milestones
- School history, including special education versus regular education, any special accommodations, and schools attended
- Social history of the family and the patient, including interactions with others, friendships, intimate relationships, and separations
- Medical history, medications, and allergies
- Drug use history
- Legal history, including who has custody and guardianship of the child
- Mental status examination of the patient, which is a description of the appearance, level of engagement, behaviors, speech, mood and affect, and thought process and content of the patient, in addition to insight and judgment

In order to be able to get all of this information, the psychiatric team has to interview the patient, the parents or guardians, the referring source, school staff, therapists, or any outpatient providers or professionals involved with the patient (Martini 2010). The task sounds simple and straightforward, but there are many limitations to this process. Not all parties can be available during the short period of time the patient is in the ER. The information received from different parties can be contradictory, or if the guardians are not the biological parents they might not know much about the history of the patient. As we said earlier, the staff has to make decisions at times without all the required information. Skilled staff can maximize the amount of information by observing subtleties of behaviors and interactions between patients and their companions, guardians, and staff. The way the patient walks into the ER, the way he sits in the waiting area, his interactions with others, his responses when asked by staff to accompany them to a different office, and his responses to questioning by staff members all inform our understanding of the case. Body language and nonverbal communication, such as attitude, eye contact, proximity to and distance from others, distractions, and facial expressions, can give us substantial clinical information. The staff can see the patient's level of impulse control, anger, sadness, and reality testing before they even start the interview or obtain basic information about the patient. Lack of impulse control, angry or intense eye contact, or a high tone of voice can alert the staff and predict a potentially dangerous situation or an angry outburst. Skilled staff can develop what we identify as the "blink phenomenon" (Gladwell 2005). Many times staff are able to formulate an opinion about the patient, especially related to predicting an explosive interaction or dangerous situation, within a few seconds of meeting the patient. Such predictions are based not on a "gut feeling" only but on clinical information gathered within seconds by close observation and years of experience.

Patients arrive at the ER in crisis. The crisis can be due to a home situation or can cause a high stress level among family members. Parents are very worried about their child, plus they have been asked to leave their jobs or home to come to the ER to be with their child and may be worried about other children at home, about problems at work, or even about losing their job. Parents may also fear that the child will be hospitalized or taken away by child protection. They may feel anger toward the referring person who was not able to manage the crisis without sending the child to the hospital and/or anger at the mental health system that did not help them before things became a crisis. In addition, many parents are worried about the stigma of being in the hospital for mental health reasons or may be entirely opposed to mental health intervention or medications. Managing a parent's anxiety and containing his or her anger can be very challenging. The staff has to connect with the parents and form an alliance in order to be able to receive the information needed for the evaluation and to provide the help necessary in each situation. Empathy, respectful listening and being able to manage anger outbursts by providing clear and honest information can help parents feel the staff will work with them and not against them. Staff should address parents' concerns head-on, reassuring the parents that their child is not going to be taken away from them (and being honest with them if in fact Child Protective Services is being called) and explaining that no medications will be prescribed without their permission. Providing clear guidelines for parents and explaining how the evaluation process is going to work can help parents manage the anxiety and their expectations. As ER providers, we must build an alliance with the family and make them part of the treatment team, because they will be responsible for carrying out the treatment plan, ensuring the child gets to follow-up appointments, and managing future crises.

Working With Emergency Room Staff

If you send a child to the ER, communication and coordination are crucial to getting the best care for the child. First, communicating with the parents is key. Before you send a child to the ER, either from a school setting or from any outpatient office or program, the parent or guardian should be informed. Explaining to the parent clearly what has happened and all the efforts you have made to de-escalate the situation will help the parent understand why a trip to the ER was needed and why it is so important that he or she drop everything to address this crisis. Communication with the

ER staff is also crucial. You know the child better than any ER physician, and the child is unlikely to truly open up to a random stranger he or she is meeting in the ER for the first time, even if (and perhaps especially because) that person is a doctor. If you are sending a child to the ER, you should relay what you know to the clinical staff there either by initiating a phone call to the ER staff or by providing a written document that includes as many details of the incident and past psychiatric history, and as much psychosocial information, as possible. This information could be crucial in determining the treatment plan, including admitting or discharging the patient. If possible, give the ER staff a phone number to call you if they have questions and to make sure you are in agreement with the treatment plan they work out.

Avoiding the Emergency Room

If you are not sure a visit to the ER is needed, taking some steps to assess and stabilize the situation onsite at your office, school, or program can be helpful in many ways. You might avert an unnecessary ER trip, and even if the child still needs to go to the ER, the way you manage the crisis helps the child feel safe with you, helps you learn about how to prevent future crises with this child, and helps you gather important information that can help the ER team make the right treatment plan.

A majority of children referred to the ER with mental health problems are discharged within the same day, suggesting that many of these kids may not have needed to go to the ER. Taking a few steps to avert or to stabilize a crisis, such as those listed below, may let you avoid an ER visit and get the child connected to the right services in other ways:

* Get familiar with the resources available in your community and in your program to manage a crisis. This will give you a sense of safety and security and will make you more able to manage a crisis should it arise. Things to think about include what mental health and social services are available in the community, and whether there are family stabilization or crisis resources, school-based mental health clinics, or family resource centers available. You should also think about your own program, both the physical space (which areas are safe and quiet) and the staff (how to call for help, how many staff are available to help with an agitated child, and which staff know the children best or have expertise in crisis situations).
* Work with your team to plan for managing a crisis. Such planning can include having available names of staff members to call for help, pro-

viding guidance for approaching the child, and determining effective interventions based on previous experiences. Having a protocol is important for staff members. Crisis means chaos, and planned procedures and interventions minimize the chaotic events.

- When you have a child with a mental health crisis, approach the child in a caring, inquisitive way rather than in a disciplinary way. The abused child, the anxious or depressed child, or the psychotic child will not respond to any disciplinary approach at the time of crisis. Their behaviors during the crisis stem from a much deeper level of fear, anger, and helplessness. In order to de-escalate the situation, you have to ensure that the child feels safe, heard, and understood. In the chaos of crisis, it all can be very blurry, and this can add to the child's fear and reactions to the surroundings.
- Know the child and the environment he or she is coming from. Being familiar with the child's background can help tremendously in understanding his or her reactions and problematic behaviors.
- Know that children in general do not want to be "in trouble" and that if they are in crisis, it is generally because they do not know how to help themselves with whatever is going on. Assuring the child in crisis that you want to help and that you want to try to find a solution can be a very helpful start. Being sincere and caring can be your key to starting a dialogue rather than getting into a screaming battle.
- Whenever staff feel that they are stuck and that there is no way around the problem, try to put yourself in the child's shoes. This can help you to understand the feelings of vulnerability and powerlessness that the child in crisis is likely feeling. Approaching the vulnerability, rather than just seeing the anger or the negative behavior, will go far to de-escalate the situation and avoid a crisis.

In This Volume

Being able to differentiate between crisis and emergency and de-escalate the situation, and being fully aware of the resources in the community, could prevent a visit to the ER in time of crisis. And knowing how best to work with the ER staff if a trip to the hospital is needed can help to ensure the children in your care get the help they need.

In this volume, we identify a range of common crisis situations, from aggressive outbursts to suicidal behaviors to possible psychosis to drug use. Each chapter identifies one of these crises; lays out some guidelines for understanding and assessing the crisis; presents a differential diagnosis of psychiatric disorders that might contribute to this type of crisis; and gives a plan for de-escalating the crisis, deciding when to go to the ER, and preventing future crises. We hope that this volume will be useful to you both in preparing for and preventing crises with the children you see and in the moment of a crisis to determine the best course of action. With the tools in this book, we hope that we can all do a better job of identifying kids at risk, getting them the help they need, and generally making our programs a safe place for our children to thrive.

References

Gladwell M: Blink: The Power of Thinking Without Thinking. New York, Little, Brown, 2005

Janssens A, Hayen S, Walraven V, et al: Emergency psychiatric care for children and adolescents: a literature review. Pediatr Emerg Care 29(9):1041–1050, 2013

Levine BH, Najara JE: Child and adolescent emergency psychiatry, in Clinical Manual of Emergency Psychiatry. Edited by Riba MB, Ravindranath D. Washington, DC, American Psychiatric Publishing, 2010, pp 207–232

Martini DR: Psychiatric emergencies, in Dulcan's Textbook of Child and Adolescent Psychiatry. Edited by Dulcan M. Washington, DC, American Psychiatric Publishing, 2010, pp 583–594

Perou R, Bitsko RH, Blumberg SJ, et al: Mental health surveillance among children—United States, 2005–2011. MMWR Surveill Summ 62 (suppl 2)1–35, 2013. Available at: http://www.cdc.gov/mmwr/preview/mmwrhtml/su6202a1.htm. Accessed May 5, 2014.

Pittsenbarger ZE, Mannix R: Trends in pediatric visits to the emergency department for psychiatric illnesses. Acad Emerg Med 21(1):25–30, 2014

Thomas LE: Trends and shifting ecologies: Part I. Child Adolesc Psychiatr Clin N Am 12(4):599–611, 2003

CHAPTER 2

Aggression

Ruth Gerson, M.D.
Fadi Haddad, M.D.

Explosive temper outbursts, verbally and physically aggressive behaviors, and violence are common occurrences in schools across the country. These behaviors are some of the most common reasons for referral to emergency psychiatric services. Aggression can be profoundly disruptive in classrooms and for families. It can be frightening to peers, teachers, and siblings and parents and in some cases can be acutely dangerous. If aggressive behaviors are persistent, the child may face suspension or expulsion from school, conflict with or exclusion by peers, family conflict leading to divorce or out-of-home placement, and even criminal charges.

Responding to aggressive behaviors in the classroom or community requires calm, clearheaded thinking, careful risk assessment, and quick action to ensure safety of the aggressive child and anyone around him or her. Although safety is the first priority, it is possible to respond to aggressive behaviors in a way that lets you learn from the crisis, to better understand the child and prevent future aggression. Aggression can often seem unpredictable or unprovoked, but there is always a reason for it. If we can identify risk factors or triggers for the aggressive behavior, we can reframe aggressive outbursts as an opportunity for learning and for helping the aggressive child get the help he or she needs.

Case Presentation

Derrick, a sixth grader in regular education, becomes disruptive in his English class, shouting that Alex, the student seated next to him, has taken his pen. As Alex denies it, Derrick begins pushing Alex, shouting, and grabbing Alex's things. The teacher tells Derrick to calm down and then takes Derrick's arm to escort him to the principal's office. At that point Derrick loses it, cursing at the teacher and struggling to get away. The school peace officer helps to escort Derrick to the principal's office, where Derrick is argumentative and disrespectful, refusing to listen to the principal or take any responsibility for his actions. When the principal tells Derrick he is suspended, Derrick really loses control, throwing books and objects from the principal's desk onto the floor, cursing and making verbal threats, and finally trying to hit the peace officer. A call was made to 911.

Understanding the Crisis

When you are dealing with aggressive behaviors, it is important to have a framework for understanding where aggression comes from and how to differentiate type and severity of aggression, as such an understanding is critical in risk assessment, de-escalation, and prevention.

Clinicians often categorize aggression as being verbal, physical, or involving destruction of property. Although these categories are useful descriptions, anyone who has worked with an aggressive child knows that most kids who are aggressive engage in all three types of aggression in some form or another. A child may start out with verbal threats, escalate to ripping up papers and breaking things in the room, and finally start kicking and hitting. A more useful way of categorizing aggressive behavior is the distinction between **reactive** and **instrumental** aggression. Aggressive behaviors, like all other behaviors, are either a reaction to something or a means to an end. When aggression is in reaction to something (e.g., a child who is being verbally teased hits back), we call it *reactive aggression,* and when aggression is a way to try to get or communicate something (e.g., a child who wants a toy hits a peer to get it), it is referred to as *instrumental aggression.* When a child engages in an aggressive act—be it a verbal threat, destruction of property, physical aggression, assault, or use of a weapon—it is either in reaction to something or an attempt to get something or communicate something. The distinction between reactive and instrumental aggression is critical in understanding and responding to aggressive behaviors.

It is also crucial to understand the context of the aggressive behavior. Is it an isolated incident or part of a pattern of aggressive behaviors or bullying? The context can also elucidate the trigger for an act of reactive aggression or the goal of an act of instrumental aggression. In the case example above, Derrick's behavior appears to be reactive, first in response to Alex's taking his pen (or Derrick's perception or belief that Alex took his pen, whether or not Alex had actually done so), then in response to the teacher's putting his hands on Derrick's arm, then in response to the principal's setting a consequence (i.e., suspension). (This type of aggression should be contrasted with instrumental aggressive acts, such as if Derrick had hit Alex in order to take his cellphone or had made threats in the classroom in order to be sent out of the class and escape an assignment that was too difficult for him.) We do not know about other contextual factors that may have contributed to the aggressive behavior. Had there been previous conflicts between Derrick and Alex or between Derrick and the teacher? Does Derrick have a history of psychiatric illness, cognitive limitations, or learning disability that may make him more likely to react with aggression? Were there any recent stressors in Derrick's life, such as parental divorce or domestic violence? Were there any prior experiences that are influencing Derrick's reactions, such as experiences of physical abuse that lead him to react violently when he is touched?

Understanding how the incident unfolded can also help us know how to help Derrick de-escalate. For example, were there any signs before this incident that Derrick was on edge or upset? How did the teacher approach Derrick? Did she empathize with Derrick's concerns or use an angry or frightened tone to immediately demand that Derrick calm down? Did she ask Derrick to leave the classroom before touching him? What were the other children in the classroom doing? How did the peace officer and principal approach Derrick? The more we know about Derrick and about the context of the aggression, the better able we will be to help him de-escalate in this moment and also prevent incidents from escalating to this level.

Identifying Kids at Risk for Aggressive Behaviors

It will come as a surprise to some (though not to those with young children) that the most aggressive period of a person's life is ages 2–3 years. As one expert in childhood aggression famously quipped, "Babies do not kill each other, because we do not give them access to knives and guns" (Holden 2000). Although almost half of toddler-age boys and slightly fewer toddler-age girls engage regularly in hitting, kicking, biting, and other aggression (Holden 2000), aggressive behaviors become less frequent as children grow; however, these behaviors can become more serious as children become both larger and more sophisticated. **Age** can be a risk factor for different types of aggression, with young children being more vulnerable to impulsive, reactive aggression (ranging from tantrums to verbal threats to physical aggression or property destruction) and older adolescents being more likely to engage in instrumental aggressive acts such as bullying or gang-related aggression. It is important not to be swayed by the child's physical appearance or even his or her age, because it is the **level of cognitive functioning** and **intellectual age** that truly determine violence risk. A child with an unrecognized intellectual disability (even a mild one), who has been held back in school or who is in a classroom that is beyond his ability, may be more likely to react with aggression when frustrated or provoked. This child is likely chronically frustrated and anxious in the classroom, which makes him vulnerable to outbursts, and also lacks the cognitive and verbal skills to identify alternative responses or ways to get what he needs. Even a child whose intellectual disability is known and who is in an appropriate school placement may still be vulnerable to outbursts if adults underestimate his limitations and expect greater maturity and ability than he can muster. Such a child might also be teased or bullied because of his disability, or older peers might take advantage of the child's lack of understanding of consequences and push him to engage in disruptive behaviors or instrumental violence.

Learning disabilities can also put children at risk for aggressive acting out. Any child whose learning disability is unrecognized or not sufficiently supported in the classroom may be chronically frustrated, feel inferior or embarrassed, or experience teasing by peers that make her vulnerable to reacting with aggression to otherwise minor provocations. A child with a specific disability in expressive language may have difficulty voicing her needs and solving problems through verbal negotiation, and so may be more likely to become frustrated and agitated at home or in the classroom. Such a child may also be more vulnerable to instrumental aggression. For example, she may hit an irritating classmate to make him stop because she is not able to voice her frustration to the teacher. Alternatively, she may begin yelling and throwing objects in order to leave the classroom if she feels overwhelmed but lacks the skills to voice her need for a break. A child with disabilities in receptive language may not be following classroom instructions (which she did not understand because of her learning disability) and then, when a consequence is set for not listening, become angry and aggressive because she does not understand why she is being punished. Children with social skills deficits, deficits in frustration tolerance or cognitive flexibility, and deficits in emotion regulation skills may also be vulnerable to aggressive behavior for similar reasons (Greene 2010).

Other chronic factors may predispose a child to aggressive behaviors, including **environmental factors** at home and at school. Children growing up in **communities with frequent violence or gang presence,** and children who witness **domestic violence** at home, may learn that aggression is an effective and appropriate means to an end. Similarly children who experience **abuse or neglect** at home are at chronically increased risk for aggression, for multiple reasons. First, abuse and neglect lead to a chronic stress response, so children's fight-or-flight response is constantly keyed up. Children who have been abused or neglected also learn to expect hostility, violence, or abuse from others, because this is what they experience at home. Finally, child abuse can lead to a lack of development of impulse control and emotion regulation skills. These factors combined make abused children more vulnerable to perceiving threats in their environment. They can perceive a threat even when there is none and react with aggression to minor provocations, such as Derrick's response when the teacher put her hand on his arm to guide him out of the classroom. A child who is being abused at home may also be irritable due to something as simple as **lack of sleep** (if the child is afraid to sleep at night or has nightmares) or **hunger** (if the child is also being neglected). Although it is important to monitor aggressive kids for signs of abuse or neglect, a child's aggressive behavior does not necessarily suggest that abuse is happening at home. Even more mild forms of stress at home can increase a child's risk of violence. Conflict between parents, parental divorce, the birth of a new sibling, or a parent's or sibling's illness may increase a child's level of stress and anxiety and make him or her vulnerable to outbursts.

The school environment can also put a child at risk for aggressive behavior. **Overcrowded classrooms** can be overwhelming and overstimulating to some children. Children who are vulnerable to explosive outbursts for whatever reason may be teased by peers because their explosions provide an amusing disruption to the classroom activity. These children are often bullied by peers, particularly if they also have cognitive limitations, learning disabilities, or mental illness. Although teachers and administrators may perceive an aggressive child as a bully, it is often the case that the child is being provoked by constant verbal bullying by more socially sophisticated peers. Adults tend to take physical bullying seriously but often underestimate the effects of **verbal bullying, cyberbullying, or relational aggression** (which involves bullying through social exclusion, social manipulation, and so forth) (Harel-Fisch et al. 2011). These types of bullying are more subtle than physical bullying but just as damaging, if not more so. When a child engages in aggressive behavior at school, it is crucial to consider whether teasing or bullying may have contributed to the behavior, because if the bullying is not addressed, the child is likely to become aggressive again regardless of the consequences set.

Finally, **psychiatric illness**, including chronic disorders such as autism spectrum disorder or attention-deficit/hyperactivity disorder (ADHD) and acute disturbances such as mania or psychosis, can put a child at risk for aggressive behaviors. It is important to remember, though, that psychiatric illness alone rarely leads to violence. Often youths with psychiatric illness are also victims of abuse, neglect, bullying, or the other stressors described in this section. It is necessary to look beyond diagnosis at the whole picture to determine how best to help an aggressive child.

Differential Diagnosis

Aggressive behavior in children should be a red flag not only for the risk factors described in the previous section but also for undiagnosed psychiatric disorder. If a child with a known mental illness has an aggressive outburst, your knowledge of the child's mental illness can guide you toward more effective de-escalation and prevention strategy. If an aggressive child does not have a known mental illness and none of the risk factors described earlier are present, a psychiatric evaluation may be indicated (see section "When to Get Help" for a discussion of when to refer for such an evaluation). Your observations and description of the aggressive outburst and any other insights into the child's behavior will be incredibly valuable to the clinician conducting the evaluation and may be a key factor in guiding him or her to the correct diagnosis.

Autism Spectrum Disorder

Children with autism spectrum disorder and other developmental disabilities can be at increased risk for aggressive behaviors for a number of reasons. Lack of verbal ability is a major risk factor for aggression. Just as toddlers have tantrums when their desires and emotions outstrip their capacity for verbal expression, autistic children without language or with delays in verbal expression may similarly engage in aggressive behavior to express frustration, anxiety, or desire to escape a stressor or sensory overstimulation. The cognitive rigidity and difficulty with transitions can also make autistic children prone to agitation. This can manifest as aggression during changes in routine, particularly if the change was not predicted in advance. Children with autism are vulnerable to teasing and bullying by peers. Sometimes they are blissfully ignorant of this due to their misperception of social cues, but many autistic children do understand then they are being teased or excluded by peers. This recognition can be extremely frustrating and hurtful and can trigger aggressive outbursts—either reactive aggression in the moment or more serious acts such as bringing a weapon to school—if the autistic child feels this is the only way to make the bullying stop. Finally, children with autism may be vulnerable to the negative influence of peers and engage in aggressive behaviors in an attempt to fit in or curry favor with peers, if they are unable to make friends in other ways.

Identifying triggers for aggressive behaviors in children with autism can be difficult, because their language deficits can make it difficult for these children to identify what set them off. Aggressive outbursts may appear to occur out of nowhere, when in fact they may have been triggered by hunger, sensory overstimulation by a clothing item or noise in the classroom, difficulty with a peer, or feelings of being overwhelmed by classwork. A careful behavioral analysis of the event can be critical in elucidating the chronic risk factors and immediate triggers, so that a behavioral plan can be put into place to avoid future outbursts. Adults are also often distressed if children with a pervasive developmental disorder do not express remorse after an aggressive act. It is important to remember that youths with autism do not perceive and understand others' emotions in the same way that neurotypical children do. They may not understand the effects of their actions on others, may laugh in anxiety when others are crying, and may need special help to understand how their aggression can harm others.

It is also important to remember that autistic disorders fall on a spectrum. Whereas some children have a more severe form of the disorder that is diagnosed at a young age, more subtle disabilities may be missed by pediatricians and psychologists. Children with average or above-average IQ and without clear language deficits may reach adolescence or young adulthood before being diagnosed. If a child in your classroom or clinic demonstrates a persistent pattern of aggressive outbursts during transitions or disruptions to routine, and also demonstrates odd or delayed use of language, poor social skills, rigidity, or unusual interests, it may be worthwhile to have him or her evaluated for an autism spectrum disorder.

Attention-Deficit/Hyperactivity Disorder

While aggression is not a core symptom of ADHD, children with ADHD are at increased risk for outbursts and aggressive behaviors related to their core symptoms of impulsivity and poor self-control. Although ADHD is generally perceived as a lack of attention, it is actually a broader syndrome of poor self-regulation, involving deficits in management of attention (with too little attention to some things, like classwork, and too much attention to others, such as video games or favorite books), poor impulse control, deficits in executive function skills (time management, organization and planning), and deficits in emotion regulation skills. Children with ADHD can be thought of as lagging 2–3 years behind their peers in the development of self-regulation skills, and these core deficits (particularly impulsivity, poor emotion regulation, and low frustration tolerance) can lead directly to aggressive outbursts. Aggressive behaviors in children with ADHD can be reactive (rooted in frustration about having to wait their turn or anger after a verbal conflict with a classmate) or instrumental (a child who "acts before he thinks" and hits a peer in order to get the other child's toy or game). Children with ADHD are at further increased risk for aggressive behaviors if they are teased or shunned by peers, who are often intolerant of their impulsivity and annoying behaviors. Children with ADHD may also be more prone to harsh discipline or physical abuse at home. Many children with ADHD have comorbid learning disabilities, which can make them prone to aggression for the reasons described above. Others, particularly if they do not receive appropriate treatment, can develop low self-esteem related to their academic and social difficulties and are then vulnerable to depression, anxiety, and substance abuse.

When a child with ADHD engages in aggressive behavior, it can be easy to attribute it solely to the symptoms of the disorder and miss other vulnerability factors such as comorbid mood problems or learning disabilities, teasing or bullying at school, or problems at home. As with autism, the evaluation and treatment of an aggressive child with ADHD will be vastly more effective if the child's clinician is made aware of triggers and contextual factors related to the child's outbursts.

Oppositional Defiant Disorder and Conduct Disorder

Frequently comorbid with ADHD but at times occurring in isolation, oppositional defiant disorder (ODD) affects as many as one in five children. Frequent tantrums and a quick temper are core symptoms of ODD, and aggressive behaviors in ODD can be both reactive (tantrums) and instrumental (purposeful aggression) in nature. Research suggests that children with ODD are more likely to feel that aggression and property destruction are justified to manage social problems with peers and adults. These behaviors often trigger anger and hostility from peers and adults, which may reinforce these maladaptive beliefs and prevent their development of alternative skills for solving problems. Children with ODD are also less aware of the impact of their aggressive behaviors on others. That is not to say that all children with ODD lack empathy and are destined for sociopathy. Although a small number of children with ODD go on to develop conduct disorder (CD) and then antisocial personality disorder (an adult psychiatric disorder characterized by aggression and lack of empathy), ODD is actually highly treatable with behavioral family interventions such as parent training or collaborative problem solving.

Many youths diagnosed with ODD have comorbid conditions, such as ADHD or depression, that also need treatment. Alternatively, children may be misdiagnosed with ODD when their aggressive behaviors in fact stem from anxiety or trauma. In youths with ODD and CD, there is often a history of abuse or severe trauma. Some estimate that as many as 50% of youths who commit crimes have a history of childhood trauma and post-traumatic stress disorder (PTSD) (Mahoney et al. 2004). In studies of juvenile criminal offenders, the severity of PTSD symptoms predicts a higher degree of delinquent behaviors (Becker and Kerig 2011; Smith and Thornberry 1995). While youths with CD can engage in very aggressive behaviors, drug use, and even gang involvement, CD too is treatable with intensive family therapy, particularly multisystemic therapy and family-focused therapy. It is also crucial to treat PTSD if it is comorbid with CD, and close observation of aggressive behaviors in youths with CD can be instrumental in identifying trauma triggers that must be addressed in treatment.

Mood and Anxiety Disorders

Mood and anxiety disorders are a spectrum of illnesses that include depressive disorders, bipolar disorder, generalized anxiety disorder, separation anxiety disorder, and panic disorder. Many of these can increase risk for aggressive behaviors, so we will examine each in turn below.

Because depression and anxiety in children and adolescents often manifests as irritability, many youths with mood and anxiety disorders are misdiagnosed as having ODD or their symptoms are missed altogether and dismissed as the "normal moodiness of adolescence." Symptoms of depression and anxiety can be very different in children and adolescents than in adults, and may contribute to aggressive behaviors. Children with depression are often irritable, with low frustration tolerance, social isolation, lack of pleasure, chronic fatigue due to poor sleep, and hopelessness that may present as lack of attention to consequences. Although these children rarely present with instrumental aggression, they may become agitated or destroy property in response to frustration and feelings of hopelessness. For others, aggressive behavior is a form of self-harm, as when they act out toward a larger peer or police and hope the target of their aggression will strike back.

Adolescents with bipolar disorder may also act out in this way, as a result of irritability or grandiosity combined with the poor judgment that characterizes mania. A third subset of children with mood disorders present with chronic negative mood, irritability, and frequent temper outbursts and are diagnosed with disruptive mood dysregulation disorder. This relatively new disorder is not well characterized but involves frequent (multiple times per week) episodes of verbal or physical aggression or destruction of property starting before the age of 10 in children whose symptoms do not meet criteria for either depression or bipolar disorder (American Psychiatric Association 2013). While treatments have not yet been developed for this disorder, close collaboration among parents, schools, and treatment providers is necessary to elucidate triggers for outbursts and guide therapy.

Children with anxiety disorders can also present with aggressive behaviors. In these cases children are not aggressive with the purpose of harming others, but may explode because of the tension caused by their fear or worry.

Obsessive-Compulsive Disorder

Children with obsessive-compulsive disorder (OCD) can also present with aggressive behaviors. As with children with anxiety disorders, children with OCD are not aggressive with the purpose of harming others, but may explode as a result of the tension caused by their fear or worry. Children with OCD may have intrusive thoughts about harming others or breaking things, or may have compulsive behaviors that when disrupted lead to outbursts. Children with OCD may have poor insight into their symptoms (an important difference between pediatric and adult OCD), so collateral information from adults who witness these outbursts at home or at school can be crucial for treatment providers.

Trauma and Posttraumatic Stress Disorder

Although depression and PTSD are the most common psychiatric consequences of childhood trauma or abuse, traumatized children can also demonstrate aggression and violence. For some, the aggression and violence are rooted in depressive, anxiety, or obsessive-compulsive symptoms as described earlier, but many traumatized youths can engage in aggressive or dysregulated behaviors even in the absence of clear mood or anxiety symptoms. In a large school-based study, each traumatic event experienced by a child increased the risk of aggressive behaviors (including physical fighting, bullying, dating violence, and bringing of weapons to school) in an additive manner from 35% to 144% (Duke et al. 2010). Abuse in childhood is associated with a 53% risk of any arrest in adolescence and with a 38% increased risk of arrest for violent crime (Widom 1992), and early abuse (before age 6) increases risk for arrest and violent crime, even after socioeconomic status, family functioning, and child's temperament are controlled for (Lansford et al. 2007). Physical abuse and witnessing of domestic violence are particularly strong predictors of aggressive behavior (Duke et al. 2010; McCabe et al. 2005; Turner et al. 2006).

If a child has been physically abused or exposed to domestic violence at home, he may learn that physical aggression is an appropriate way to solve problems or respond to conflict (Cullerton-Sen et al. 2008). But other children who have experienced trauma may become aggressive because of trauma reminders. For example, some children who have been abused may become aggressive when touched by a peer or adult even in a benign way, because the touch of another person triggers reminders of their abuse. Other children may react with aggression to sudden loud noises, if the noises remind them of gunshots or of their mother screaming because she is being beaten by her drunk boyfriend. Children who have experienced home invasions or school shootings may react violently to school safety drills, which may trigger reminders or flashbacks of their earlier experience. PTSD can further increase a traumatized child's risk for aggression, and for reactive aggression in particular. The hypervigilance and flashbacks of PTSD can lead a child to overreact to minor provocations or to become lost in a flashback and fight back against an absent but perceived attacker. After these outbursts, most children say they cannot remember what they said or did or what triggered their behavior. They are not avoiding responsibility; they may truly be unable to remember. Trauma reminders can have a profound impact on memory and cognition, leading to confusion or even dissociated states. If a child becomes aggressive apparently out of nowhere and afterward seems dazed or unable to recall the event, a possible history of trauma or abuse should be considered.

Psychosis

Psychosis can manifest as part of many psychiatric syndromes, including depression, mania, and schizophrenia. Psychosis is defined by a confusion between real events and unreal ones. Individuals with psychosis may become aggressive in response to internal stimuli such as hallucinations or delusions or in response to misperceptions of others' behavior. While many individuals with psychosis are never aggressive, certain symptoms, such as paranoia and command auditory hallucinations, are predictive of violence risk. Psychosis is extremely rare in children and uncommon in adolescents, however, and aggression is rarely the first symptom. Most adolescents with psychosis present first with symptoms such as social isolation, withdrawal from activities, academic deterioration, odd behaviors, lack of emotions, and odd speech and thinking. Many children will endorse hearing or seeing things when asked, but this does not necessarily represent psychosis and may be age-appropriate (such as imaginary friends) or a way of trying to avoid responsibility for their actions (e.g., a young child saying that a voice told him to hit his classmate).

Substance Use

Although rare in children, experimentation with drugs and alcohol is common in adolescents. Different drugs and alcohol vary in their effect on the brain and can have different immediate effects during intoxication and delayed effects during withdrawal or drug-seeking behaviors. An adolescent may be agitated and irritable because of intoxication with cocaine or phencyclidine (PCP), or during alcohol or opiate withdrawal, or can be agitated because of the psychological need for the drug. Gang involvement is not uncommon in these scenarios, and related aggressive or criminal behaviors may spill over into incidents at school.

Identifying Immediate Triggers

While identifying chronic risk factors and possible psychiatric contributors to aggressive behavior (Table 2–1), as noted earlier in this chapter, it is also critical to observe any **immediate triggers** and ascertain how chronic or internal risk factors may be set off by events in the social environment or classroom (Minahan and Rappaport 2012). For example, a child with ADHD and depression who is struggling with poverty at home and is often hungry may be teased by peers for her appearance. If she explodes, this may reinforce the peers' bullying, as her explosion provides a welcome and perhaps amusing distraction from schoolwork. An autistic child may explode because he is overwhelmed by the noise in the classroom, and an abused child may explode because she sees a man who looks like the stepfather who abused her. It is also important to consider the experience from the **child's perspective.** If a child engages in instrumental aggression, does he feel his behavior was justified, or does he lack the skills to get his needs met in other ways? When a child engages in reactive aggression, it is important to recognize that most children, when acutely dysregulated, lose language skills: there is literally less blood flow to language centers of the brain during emotional dyregulation in children. These children are often frightened by and ashamed of their loss of control, and they may need special support and interventions while they build skills to solve problems more effectively.

Risk Assessment

The most important and first step in helping any child in crisis is **risk assessment.** For an aggressive child, it is critical to maintain the safety of the child and any surrounding children and adults. Assessment of the child is

TABLE 2–1. Risk factors and immediate triggers for aggressive behavior

Environmental factors	Community violence
	Domestic violence
	Physical abuse or neglect
	Bullying or cyberbullying
	Overcrowded classroom
Child factors	Unrecognized learning disability
	Young age
	Intellectual disability
Psychiatric illness	Autism spectrum disorder
	Attention-deficit/hyperactivity disorder
	Oppositional defiant disorder or conduct disorder
	Anxiety disorders (generalized anxiety disorder, separation anxiety disorder, panic disorder)
	Obsessive-compulsive disorder
	Mood disorders (depression, bipolar disorder)
	Psychosis
	Trauma and posttraumatic stress disorder
	Substance use
Immediate triggers	Teasing by peers
	Classwork that is too difficult
	Hunger or pain
	Reminders of traumatic experiences or abuse
	Fear or anxiety
	Overstimulation (particularly for kids with autism)

important, but even before that, the **environment** must be considered. Is the child in a crowded area with many other children and few adults? Peers can be frightened or injured if they are nearby. Alternatively, peers might laugh and egg a child on, which can further exacerbate an agitated child's anger or anxiety. Is the aggressive child in a room with sharp or heavy objects that could be used as a weapon or thrown at others? Moving others out of the area and removing any potentially dangerous objects is a crucial first step, and should be followed by gathering additional trusted adults for support. Neither the child nor the staff can work toward de-escalation if they are not in a safe space.

After the environment is observed, the child's **history** should be considered. A child with a known history of severe aggression or assault will be more concerning than a child who has no history of aggression or who has frequent tantrums but can calm down quickly. If there are individuals or stimuli that are known to trigger aggression in the child (e.g., a certain noise in an autistic child, or a threatening figure in a traumatized child) and that can be easily removed, this also suggests that de-escalation may be possible. The age and size of the child will also influence whether the child can be contained onsite by a few adults or whether professional backup is needed.

Finally, consider the child's **current behavior.** Is he agitated, verbally threatening, breaking objects, or hitting others or brandishing a weapon? The severity of current aggression should be considered in determining whether peace officers, emergency medical services (EMS), or police should be called. The nature of the aggression also dictates the response. If the aggression is clearly instrumental and premeditated, without provocation, then the police and legal system should be involved to avoid further assaults and injuries and to set appropriate consequences. If the aggression is reactive or related to psychiatric illness, consider eliciting help from the school psychologist or EMS. They can assist in stabilization, identifying triggers, and developing a treatment plan. Also consider the child's response to your efforts at stabilization. If the child is able to respond to verbal reassurance and interventions as described below, she is at lower risk than if she were in the midst of a flashback, not making sense, or appearing to be experiencing command auditory hallucinations. A quick appraisal of the child will guide you in your approach to stabilization and de-escalation.

Onsite Stabilization

Even if you have already decided to call 911 or police, de-escalating the crisis onsite as much as possible is important. De-escalation can prevent injury and assault and minimize the negative impact on both the child in crisis and any adults and children witnessing the event. The process of de-escalation is complex and requires close collaboration and trust among the adults involved. One person should be identified as the leader of the de-escalation process, preferably someone who has a positive relationship with the child. Others can focus on providing support, moving other children or dangerous objects out of the way, or calling for emergency personnel. Only one person should talk to the child at a time, or else the child can become overwhelmed and more aggressive.

It is also critical that all adults remain calm. Children can "feel" our emotions clearly, and if they perceive that we are angry or afraid, they feel more angry and afraid. Any adult who feels angry, very frightened, or targeted by the child should remove himself or herself from the situation. Also, any adult who might be perceived by the child as threatening—for example, if he or she had a bad relationship with the child from previous interactions—should remove himself or herself and perhaps focus on redirecting and reassuring the other children in the area.

Catch the Warning Signs

The best way to deal with aggression is to catch it as early as possible, when the child is most amenable to intervention. Aggressive behaviors generally have three stages: a ramp-up, when the child is becoming more upset and agitated; a period of aggression; and then a cooling-down stage. While the ramp-up may be subtle, it is rare that a child becomes aggressive without some warning signs. Parents, teachers, or others who interact closely with the child may be able to identify these early warning signs, which could include a change in facial expression or posture, a bouncing knee or tapping pencil, a sudden negative or argumentative attitude, or withdrawal from peers. Children with autism spectrum disorder may have more idiosyncratic early warning signs of frustration or agitation, so eliciting the support of someone who knows the child well can be crucial. In the case given earlier, if the teacher had noticed signs of Derrick's frustration early on, she could have approached Derrick calmly, separated him from Alex, heard and empathized with his concerns, and either given him another pen or given him a different, "special" task to distract him.

Finding an adult who knows the child well can be extremely helpful. Simply having a trusted adult present can calm many children, particularly those who are becoming agitated because of frustration, anxiety, trauma reminders, or even psychosis. Someone who knows the child well can also give valuable information about the child's history, what has triggered outbursts for this child in the past, whether there is any history of trauma or psychiatric illness that may influence the approach to de-escalation, and what has worked in the past to calm her down. For example, a guidance counselor who knows Derrick well might have been able to tell the teacher that Derrick is sensitive to touch due to physical abuse at home, and that he is terrified about getting in trouble at school for fear his father will beat him again. With this information, the teacher and principal might have chosen different ways of calming Derrick and setting consequences for his behavior.

Listen and Empathize

Aggression is a means, not an end in itself. To help aggressive children calm down, you need to understand what it is they are trying to say or do.

Approach the child gently but assertively, from a safe distance and with a calm and soft voice. Do not yell at him or threaten consequences if he does not calm down, and do not try to distract him or make a joke. Be serious, empathic, and curious about what has happened and why the child is upset. In the case of Derrick, the teacher or a staff member who knows Derrick well might observe that he is having a hard time and express that they would like to help. Even a more neutral comment, like "Hey, you don't seem like your usual self, what happened?" can be helpful. If the child cannot say why he is upset or denies feeling upset, remain empathic and observe that his body language and behavior appear to indicate that he is upset, angry, or frustrated, and explain that you would like to help and understand. The teacher might say, "Derrick, it seems like it's hard to articulate what's going on, but I do want to help, and I'm noticing that your body looks tense. I'm guessing maybe you feel frustrated. Is that close to what you're feeling?" Make a benign observation such as that it is hard to be frustrated when no one understands, or hazard a guess if you think you know why the child is upset. Continue to stay calm and empathize as much as possible. If the child is able to identify what made him upset, reflect back what he said: "What I understand from what you are saying is that…." Validate and empathize with the child's concerns, with comments like "Wow, yeah, I can see how much that upset you" or "I can see how frustrating that would be." Do not yet try to find solutions; first make sure you completely understand what the child feels. Reflect back what he said again, and ask if there are other things that are bothering him, or other aspects that he could help you understand: "I see how that would be upsetting; are there other things or other parts that are also getting to you, or other parts I should understand?" Praise his ability to articulate a difficult situation or problem. Try to elicit his thoughts and feelings, and be radically empathic—try to take his perspective without judgment. In the process of asking him to explain, you are making it clear that you want to help, and at the same time helping him to regain cognitive control, analyze the situation, and make better choices.

Collaborate to Find Solutions

It is crucial throughout the de-escalation process to read the child's body language and constantly reevaluate your risk assessment. Is the child unclenching his fists and starting to talk to you, or is he becoming more agitated? If the child is engaging with your empathic statements and validation, you can start to work toward a solution. Summarize what he has said to you, reflecting back his feelings and emotions, and ask if you understand correctly. Offer the child some choices; for example, "I really want to help with this so I'd like to talk more; do you want to talk here or come sit down in my office?" Thank him for being willing to work on this with you, and reflect and praise any positive steps he is taking, like taking deep breaths or lowering his voice: "Thanks for coming and sitting down with me. I'm so impressed by how you're staying calm and taking those deep breaths–I know that's so hard for me to do when I get upset." You can then cautiously start to problem solve with the child, prompting him to think about his options and going over the pros and cons of each. Very gently, you can reframe and help him think through where his choices will lead. If the aggression is instrumental in nature, help him think of other ways to get what he wants. Do not give punishments, but remind the child of the consequences of his behaviors in a matter-of-fact way. If he is able to make a positive choice, praise and validate that choice and his decision to calm down and work things through.

If the child is able to calm down and problem solve with you, it is important not to jump immediately to punishment. A child who is in the cooling-down stage of a crisis is still in crisis and needs quiet, support, and positive reinforcement of his decision to calm down and of the ways he is helping himself stay calm. You are not letting him off the hook–consequences will come later–but if you start giving consequences now, he will not be able to hear them and will explode again.

It is also important to remember the impact on any children or adults who were nearby or witnessed this event. Talking with them and, while protecting the child's privacy, helping the other students to feel empathy that their classmate was having a hard time but is doing better now, can be helpful to calm the other children and repair any damage to the child's peer relationships.

Learning From the Crisis

Once the child and everyone else has fully recovered from the crisis, it can be useful to revisit the incident to learn from it and prevent a future crisis. Remembering again that aggressive behavior always happens for a reason, talk with the other adults about what they observed and remember, and then talk with the child. Ask him what his recollections are about his thoughts, feelings, and behavior during the incident, before, and after. Let him express his fear, anger, frustration, and remorse about the event. Ask about any changes, stressors, or events in his day leading up to the outburst that may help to explain it. Did he not sleep well last night? Was there tension with dad this morning? Was the classwork too stressful? Was he hungry? Did another child say something that upset him? For most children, the reasons for their behavior will not be immediately clear, even to themselves, so you may have to hazard a few guesses. By helping a child to think it through, you are helping him to develop important skills of self-awareness and self-control.

When to Get Help

If an aggressive child has been able to calm down, stay calm, and talk through the incident with you, the kind of help she needs should be informed by what you learned from that discussion. If the child revealed that a major trigger is feeling unable to keep up with classwork, then an educational evaluation may be necessary. If bullying is occurring, or the child is feeling stressed about her parents' divorce, then either the school psychologist or the guidance counselor should be involved to give her the necessary support to get through this, and the child should be referred for an outpatient psychological or psychiatric evaluation. These outpatient evaluations are much more comprehensive than one done in the emergency room (ER), and the outpatient clinician can continue to treat the child to get at the core symptoms and deficits that are at the root of the aggressive behavior. If the child has an outpatient therapist or psychiatrist already, the family should be encouraged to see that clinician within the next few days for evaluation and stabilization. That clinician will want to speak with you and the child about the incident, and the information you provide will guide the treatment plan.

If in reviewing the event, the child admits that there is abuse in the home, or that she has been depressed and has been cutting herself or having suicidal thoughts, then an ER evaluation is needed to ensure safety. Similarly, if the child cools down after an outburst but then becomes agitated again later in the day, an emergency evaluation is indicated for evaluation and safety. In these cases, parents should be called and either parents or EMS should transport the child to the hospital, and the child should be informed that this is happening. Make it clear to the child that this is not a punishment and that the goal is to understand why this happened and prevent future aggression. Be mindful that calling EMS or the police can be very frightening and even traumatic for some children, and they may feel trapped or attacked. Being transparent with the child about what is happening, the reason for calling EMS and going to the hospital, and what will happen in the evaluation can help the child feel safe and remain calm. If the child does become agitated, remember your de-escalation plan: catch the warning signs to address agitation early, listen and empathize, and collaborate to find solutions. Having a trusted staff member or parent with the child during this process can also help ease the child's fears and smooth the trip to the hospital.

If you do refer a child to the ER, remember that your observations and descriptions are critical for the ER staff to conduct an effective evaluation. A phone call and referral letter describing the child's behaviors, what was going on before the event and any stressors you identified, the child's history, her social and emotional functioning, and her academic ability will be greatly appreciated by the emergency clinicians and will help them to make the right treatment recommendations. You want to send as much information as you can (including any prior behavioral reports, educational testing, or other information that you have). By the time a child arrives in the ER, she is generally calm and often can be playful and charming as if nothing had happened. Parents who have not witnessed the event may not know what happened. Therefore, the information from the referring teacher, guidance counselor, or therapist is often some of the most useful information an emergency clinician has.

In addition to reviewing your report, the emergency clinician will take a full medical and psychiatric history from the parent, including any changes in the child's behavior or functioning, any recent or chronic stressors, prior treatments, history of medical illnesses, and family medical and psychiatric history. The clinician will also evaluate the child, assessing her ability to discuss the incident, her stressors, her insight and coping skills for managing stress, and her mental status, and also screen for any suicidal or homicidal thoughts or psychosis. The clinician may want to do a physical exam, order lab tests, and even arrange for a brain scan to assist in diagnosis. After all of this, the clinician will be able to make safety determinations and treatment recommendations. If a child is at acute risk for further aggressive behavior or for harm to herself, the clinician will likely recommend hospitalization. Most children do not need this level of care, in which case the clinician will recommend that the child and family be seen by a therapist or psychiatrist to begin treatment, which could include psychotherapy, family therapy, or medication. The ER staff should assist in finding an outpatient provider for the child. If you collaborate with the family to ensure that the child gets to that appointment and continues to engage in treatment, you can see that the child gets the help she needs to avoid aggressive outbursts in the future.

References

American Psychiatric Association: Diagnostic and Statistical Manual of Mental Disorders, 5th Edition. Arlington, VA, American Psychiatric Association, 2013

Becker SP, Kerig PK: Posttraumatic stress symptoms are associated with the frequency and severity of delinquency among detained boys. J Clin Child Adolesc Psychol 40(5):765–771, 2011

Cullerton-Sen C, Cassidy AR, Murray-Close D, et al: Childhood maltreatment and the development of relational and physical aggression: the importance of a gender-informed approach. Child Dev 79(6):1736–1751, 2008

Duke NN, Pettingell SL, McMorris BJ, Borowsky IW: Adolescent violence perpetration: associations with multiple types of adverse childhood experiences. Pediatrics 125(4):e778–e786, 2010

Greene RW: The Explosive Child: A New Approach for Understanding and Parenting Easily Frustrated, Chronically Inflexible Children. New York, Harper, 2010

Harel-Fisch Y, Walsh SD, Fogel-Grinvald H, et al: Negative school perceptions and involvement in school bullying: a universal relationship across 40 countries. J Adolesc 34(4):639–652, 2011

Holden C: The violence of the lambs. Science 289(5479):580–581, 2000

Lansford JE, Miller-Johnson S, Berlin LJ, et al: Early physical abuse and later violent delinquency: a prospective longitudinal study. Child Maltreat 12(3):233–245, 2007

Mahoney K, Ford JD, Ko SJ, et al: Trauma focused interventions for youth in the juvenile justice system. The National Child Traumatic Stress Network, 2004. Available at: http://www.nctsnet.org/nctsn_assets/pdfs/edu_materials/trauma_focused_interventions_youth_jjsys.pdf. Accessed February 10, 2014.

McCabe KM, Lucchini SE, Hough RL, et al: The relation between violence exposure and conduct problems among adolescents: a prospective study. Am J Orthopsychiatry 75:575–584, 2005

Minahan J, Rappaport N: The Behavior Code: A Practical Guide to Understanding and Teaching the Most Challenging Students. Boston, MA, Harvard Education Press, 2012

Smith C, Thornberry TP: The relationship between child maltreatment and adolescent involvement in delinquency. Criminology 33:451–481, 1995

Turner HA, Finkelhor D, Ormrod RK: The effect of lifetime victimization on the mental health of children and adolescents. Social Sci Med 62:13–27, 2006

Widom CS. The Cycle of Violence. NCJ 136607. Washington, DC, U.S. Department of Justice, National Institute of Justice, 1992

Catch the Warning Signs

1. If the child appears to be getting agitated, intervene early.
2. Recruit someone whom the child knows and trusts to help.
3. Try to understand the child's reason for getting upset.
4. Remove any instigating stressors or triggers.
5. Remove other children and any potentially dangerous objects from the area.

De-escalation: Listen and Empathize

1. Reflect, empathize, and validate the child's feelings and emotions.
2. Ask the child what is wrong, what he is feeling, and what he needs.
3. Reflect back what he tells you to make sure you understand.
4. Praise his decision to calm down and talk things through.

If the Child Continues to Be Aggressive:

1. Call for help.
2. Give the child clear and concise choices: if he calms down, you will do this; if he does not stop, this will happen.
3. If you need to, physically hold the child to prevent him from injuring himself or others, or call 911.

De-escalation: Collaborate for Solutions

1. Understand and validate the child's concerns.
2. Problem solve together, helping the child to see the pros and cons.
3. Praise the child's decision to calm down.
4. Support the child as he cools off; do not give punishment yet.

Refer to the Emergency Room if:

1. The child continues to be aggressive.
2. The child calms down but becomes agitated again later that day.
3. The child expresses suicidal or homicidal thoughts or threats.
4. The child reports that he is being abused at home.

De-escalation: Learn From the Crisis and Refer for Outpatient Treatment if:

1. You see signs of depression, anxiety, ADHD, autism, or other psychiatric diagnoses.
2. You feel the child may have unrecognized learning disabilities.
3. The child is experiencing family stress (divorce, birth of new sibling) that is upsetting him.

Managing an aggressive child in crisis.

CHAPTER 3

Suicide and Self-Injurious Behaviors

Gabrielle S. Carson, Ph.D.

Suicidal thoughts, suicide attempts, and self-injurious behaviors are serious and challenging problems in children and adolescents. Suicide is the third leading cause of death for youths ages 10–24 (Anderson and Smith 2005; Centers for Disease Control and Prevention 2007). Suicide attempts are very rare in children, though younger children can experience suicidal thoughts. Unfortunately, in an adolescent population suicide attempts are more common. Each year, 1 in 5 teenagers seriously considers suicide, and 1 in 12 actually makes a suicide attempt (Centers for Disease Control and Prevention 2012). The risk associated with suicidal thoughts or statements can be challenging to assess and poses a scary and difficult situation for schools, parents, and others who work closely with children.

The reasons a child or teen thinks about or makes a suicide attempt are varied, but generally those who make an attempt are under great stress and are unable to see a way out of their difficulties. The "last straw" that pushes a child to make a suicide attempt is often a common life stressor, such as having an argument with parents, going through a breakup of a romantic relationship, being rejected by friends, failing a class, getting a disappointing report card, or another typical childhood difficulty. Although one of these ubiquitous life challenges is often the "last straw" before a suicide attempt, those who are suicidal are usually experiencing more complicated underlying issues and almost always demonstrate warning signs that they are in trouble. Identifying these warning signs, addressing the underlying issues, and getting help for children at risk of suicide is an extremely important but often challenging undertaking.

Many children and adolescents will injure themselves without intent to die. Self-injurious behaviors, including cutting, burning, or other intentional self-injury, are problematic in and of themselves and are also indicative of an increased risk for suicide (Guan et al. 2012). Sometimes adolescents will cut or burn themselves as a suicide attempt, but more commonly children do not wish to die but are using the self-harm as an attempt to cope with emotional pain and stress. Teens often describe cutting as providing a "release" from intense and distressing emotions, or as transmuting emotional pain into physical pain that is experienced as more bearable. It is often used when teens do not have more effective ways of coping with emotional pain. Understanding the intention behind a teen's self-injurious behavior is important in assessing risk and determining ways to intervene. Regardless of the intention, self-injury is a serious problem that necessitates intervention.

Suicidality and self-injurious behaviors can be vulnerable to "copycat" effects: knowing a peer or classmate in the community who cuts or who died by suicide increases the risk for other teens in that community. Proactive intervention in these situations is crucial and can be very effective.

Case Presentation

Leila is a 15-year-old girl who is generally a good student but who recently has had a drop in her grades and has been attending school inconsistently for the past 3 weeks. Leila's teachers have noticed not only that her attendance has recently been poor but that she no longer participates much in class and has been rude and irritable with her teachers when asked questions. In addition, one of Leila's friends came to Leila's homeroom teacher to tell her that Leila had cut herself on her arm with a broken pencil and had been showing the cuts to friends and classmates. Leila became upset when the teacher inquired about her cutting and recent behavior and stated, "I can't do this anymore. Everyone should just leave me alone." The teacher expressed concern to the school guidance counselor, and Leila was then taken to the office, where she cried for the next 30 minutes and stated she wished that she "could just disappear" and that "everyone would just leave me alone and get off my back." Leila had been in therapy in the past for treatment of depression and had been prescribed an antidepressant medication but had ended treatment, and she is not currently taking any medication or receiving any counseling or therapy.

Understanding the Crisis

For parents, families, and professionals working with children and teens, the thought of a child attempting suicide is terrifying and overwhelming. Gaining as much information as possible regarding the level and type of suicidality or nonsuicidal self-injury is the first step. The Centers for Disease Control and Prevention has adopted different categories of suicidal thoughts and behaviors to help clinicians communicate clearly about risk and decide the right level of treatment. These are based on the Columbia Suicide Severity Rating Scale system of categorization (Crosby et al. 2011). The three categories for these thoughts and behaviors, listed in Table 3–1, comprise five levels of suicidal ideation and five levels of suicidal behavior, as well as a category "self-injurious behavior, no suicidal intent."

TABLE 3–1. Categories of suicidal thoughts and behaviors, adopted by the Centers for Disease Control and Prevention as defined by the Columbia Suicide Severity Rating Scale (Posner et al. 2011)

Suicidal ideation

Passive

Active, nonspecific—no method or plan

Active—method but no intent or plan

Active—method and intent but no plan

Active—method, intent, and plan

Suicidal behavior

Completed suicide

Suicide attempt

Interrupted attempt

Aborted attempt

Preparatory actions toward imminent suicidal behaviors

Self-injury, no suicidal intent

Source. Posner et al. 2011.

Suicidal ideation refers to ideas about suicide and can include thoughts or fantasies about death and dying. *Passive suicidal ideation* refers to thoughts about dying without any intent to act on these thoughts and without any plan for how one would go about committing suicide. Passive suicidal ideation includes thoughts and statements such as "I wish I didn't exist," "I'd be better off dead," or "I wish I could just not wake up in the morning." *Active suicidal ideation* includes thoughts about dying or killing oneself but with the added element of either a means for committing suicide, some intent to act on the thought, or a full plan for how the person might commit suicide.

Suicidal behavior refers to any step the person has taken toward acting on suicidal thoughts. This could include saving medication in preparation for a potential overdose, walking along the river considering places to jump in, or actually making an attempt, such as attempting to hang oneself, taking an overdose, or possibly, with younger children, running into traffic.

Self-injurious behavior such as cutting, scratching, or burning can be *suicidal* or *nonsuicidal,* and this distinction is dependent on the individual's intentions when engaging in the behavior as well as his or her understanding of the consequences of those behaviors. Often children and adolescents self-injure without any intent or desire to die (**nonsuicidal self-injury**). Reasons for this type of self-injury can include release of overwhelming emotions, an attempt to alleviate numbness and "feel something," or an expression of distress. In other cases cutting or other forms of self-injury are done with suicidal intent, and the child or teen thinks or hopes that he or she will die as a result of the injury. In these cases, the self-injury *is* considered suicidal in nature.

In the case example, Leila had engaged in self-injurious behavior and had expressed passive suicidal thoughts when she stated that she wished she "could just disappear." In understanding her case further, it is important to look closely for other warning signs and to ask the other adults that know her well about any observed changes in behavior or mood In the case example, there are signs that things have not been going well for Leila for at least a few weeks. It would be important to understand if something changed for her during this time, including new or increased stressors such as a death in the family, or if Leila was the victim of some type of traumatic event or abuse. It is possible that a falling out with a close friend, bullying, a breakup, or a parental divorce could be contributing to Leila feeling worse.

It is also important to understand what took place on the day of the cutting or during that week that led to her self-injury, and for how long Leila has been feeling this way. If Leila can describe how she was feeling and what she was thinking when she cut herself, and in the moments just before and after, it can help us understand the function of the self-injury (e.g., to relieve overwhelming emotions or anxiety). There may be factors from earlier in the day or week—even things as small as poor sleep the night before—that can make a child vulnerable to feeling overwhelmed and turning to self-harm. The way that others respond to self-harm and suicidal statements can also make a child more likely to engage in these behaviors. For example, when Leila disclosed her cutting to her friends, they likely gave her a lot of attention, concern, and reassurance. Such attention helped her feel better in the moment but in the long term may increase her likelihood of cutting again in order to get that similarly positive attention. Self-injury and suicidal statements can for some children be a way of expressing something—a need for attention or a desire for help—that they do not know how to put into words.

Any information that parents or school staff are aware of regarding previous self-injury, statements about death or suicide, suicide attempts, research Leila has done on suicide methods, or steps taken toward acting on suicidal thoughts should be clearly communicated to any outpatient mental health professional or emergency mental health team who will be evaluating Leila. In this case, Leila also has a known history of depression but is not currently being treated. This may be contributing to worsening of depression. The reasons Leila has ended treatment, whether it was helpful for her in the past, and if there has been any attempt to restart therapy or medication could be explored with Leila and her parents to add to the understanding of her recent difficulties.

Identifying Kids at Risk for Suicide

There are many varied risk factors associated with suicide, but there are also some clear warning signs. Approximately 90% of those who die from suicide have depression, other psychiatric disorders, and/or substance use disorders (Fleischmann et al. 2005). Frequently children and teens who attempt suicide have a psychiatric disorder and are simultaneously using drugs or alcohol. Taking these factors seriously and intervening quickly to address them is one of the best ways to prevent suicide.

Major depression in particular has been identified as a significant risk factor for completed suicide in adolescents. Even some depressive symptoms in the absence of a formal diagnosis put a child at increased risk for suicidality (Wolitzky-Taylor et al. 2010). In the school setting, signs of depression might include a drop in grades, inconsistent attendance, dropping out of activities, isolating from friends, crying or tearfulness, and coming to school drunk or high, as well as angry outbursts. Kids who show any combination of these risk factors should be evaluated further.

Children and adolescents who are thinking about suicide often give some indication that they are having these thoughts. This often occurs in the form of making statements about death, dying, or ending their life; writing online or in a journal about death or dying; posting messages online saying goodbye to friends and family; or giving away personal possessions. Any of these statements or behaviors is cause for concern and more thorough investigation.

Previous suicide attempts, even if they were not life threatening, are a significant and important warning sign. Children and adolescents who have made suicide attempts in the past are at higher risk for subsequent attempts and for completing suicide, even if they have been hospitalized or received treatment after that attempt (Nock et al. 2013). All suicide attempts, regardless of the lethality, type, or intention, should be taken seriously and are a clear indication that something is wrong.

Children who are under certain types of **severe stress** are at higher risk of becoming suicidal. Stressors that have been identified with increased risk of suicide include exposure to violence or trauma, including physical or sexual abuse; socioeconomic disadvantage; and identifying as gay, lesbian, bisexual, or transgender (Liu and Mustanski 2012). Having a family member who attempted or committed suicide also increases the level of risk for children within that family, particularly if the child knew the relative who committed suicide. Additionally, children and adolescents who are experiencing significant recent changes such as a change in residence, parents' divorce, breakup of their own romantic relationship, or death of a loved one may also be at increased risk. More recently, **bullying and cyberbullying** have been implicated as a significant factor in many teen suicides. Bullying causes immense distress and contributes to social isolation and feelings of worthlessness. Children who are dealing with one or more of these stressors may benefit from proactive support and intervention on the part of adults as well as careful monitoring.

Being subjected to **traumatic events,** including physical abuse, sexual abuse, or witnessing domestic or community violence, increases a child's risk of suicide (Saewyc and Chen 2013). Many traumatized children have posttraumatic stress disorder (PTSD), anxiety, depression, or behavioral problems, or are more prone to risk-taking behaviors. Children who have experienced trauma often live with a heightened level of anxiety, a feeling that the world or their surroundings are not safe, a fear of being victimized again, and feelings of shame, self-loathing, or guilt. A child who has been abused or has witnessed violence should be evaluated to determine if they have symptoms of PTSD or other symptoms that require treatment or follow-up. Good active treatment can prevent the stress associated with trauma exposure from progressing to suicidality.

Children and adolescents who are **impulsive** and take frequent risks are also at increased risk for suicide. Adolescents generally have a tendency to act impulsively without thinking through the consequences of their actions, because of the way the brain develops during adolescence, and those who are using substances or struggling with mental illness can be even more impulsive. Suicide risk is higher in teens who use alcohol or drugs, smoke cigarettes, fight physically, bring a gun to school, and are sexually active. It can be easy to dismiss problematic behavior as simply acting out and treat it as a disciplinary problem, but these behaviors should be red flags that someone is not doing well, and possible underlying causes for these behaviors–including abuse, depression, and bullying–should be examined.

Knowledge of the death of a peer in the school or community by suicide can also increase the risk of teen suicide within that community. Children and teens are vulnerable to **"copycat" attempts,** so if there is a suicide within the community, schools and community leaders should organize outreach and prevention services to identify other teens at risk.

Social media plays an increasingly powerful role in the lives of many children and teens. Often social media can provide a source of support for children that may be isolated from peers within their schools and communities, and teens at risk for suicide may use these outlets to reach out for help. At the same time, social media has also been used for bullying, and teens reaching out for help may be humiliated and harassed online and may even be encouraged by others to kill themselves. Social media has also been used by teens seeking encouragement from other teens who are suicidal. Online suicide pacts, sites where teens talk about cutting or other self-injury, and even posted videos showing methods of self-harm are increasingly common and seriously problematic. There is no substitute for careful monitoring by parents and limit setting around the use of social media if there is any indication or suspicion that any of these things are occurring.

Both boys and girls can become suicidal; however, girls have been found to have more suicidal thoughts and to have made more suicide attempts, whereas boys are more likely to actually die as a result of a suicide attempt, because they tend to choose more dangerous and violent methods (Centers for Disease Control and Prevention 2007). Finally, access to lethal means, particularly firearms, increases the risk that a child or teen will complete suicide.

Differential Diagnosis

The vast majority of children and adolescents who express suicidal thoughts, make suicidal attempts, or intentionally injure themselves have either diagnosed or undiagnosed psychiatric disorders. Suicidality should be a clear sign that something is wrong and is an indication that the child should be evaluated not only for immediate risk but also for underlying psychiatric disorders. Self-injurious behavior, while not always suicidal in nature, is also a sign that the child is unable to cope with something in his or her life in an adaptive and healthy way and also requires close monitoring and treatment.

Depression

Many suicidal children and teens have been quietly struggling with depression for some time. Depression can look different in different children but often includes noticeable changes in behavior and functioning. Symptoms of depression include sadness, irritability, loss of interest in previously enjoyed activities, feelings of guilt or worthlessness, sleep changes (including sleeping too much or too little), appetite changes, social withdrawal, and hopelessness. Some children present as much more irritable, easily frustrated, and angry when depressed. The feelings of sadness and hopelessness that often come with depression can often lead children to feel that things will never change or improve and that suicide is their only escape from pain and misery. Some children cut themselves to escape the numbness that can accompany depression or to attempt to alleviate the emotional pain of feeling depressed.

Bipolar Disorder

Bipolar disorder includes the symptoms of depression discussed above, as well as periods of mania: several days or weeks of decreased need for sleep, excessive energy, feelings of euphoria and invincibility, increased irritability, grandiosity, and risk-taking behaviors. Bipolar disorder is rare in children, and not all moodiness or mood swings in children constitute bipolar disorder. Often, in children, depressive and manic symptoms can be mixed and are less clearly divided into easily identifiable episodes than they are in adults. Emotion dysregulation, rapid changes in mood, and explosive outbursts, as well as hallucinations and delusions, can be symptoms of bipolar disorder. Bipolar disorder can increase risk for suicidality in children and teens for several reasons. First, it impairs rational thinking and makes teens more impulsive, putting them at risk for impulsive self-destructive behavior. Second, the symptoms of bipolar disorder are difficult to manage, often contribute to interpersonal problems, and can affect self-esteem. Youths newly diagnosed with bipolar disorder should be carefully monitored as they cope with the stress of their new diagnosis and of coming to terms with it.

Anxiety Disorders and Obsessive-Compulsive–Related Disorders

There are many types of anxiety disorders, including generalized anxiety disorder, panic disorder, separation anxiety, and specific and social phobias. Obsessive-compulsive disorder, once classified as an anxiety disorder but now placed in a different diagnostic class (obsessive-compulsive–related disorders), also involves marked anxiety. Excessive anxiety is a very distressing and uncomfortable experience and can be difficult to tolerate for an extended time period, so adolescents may cut themselves to relieve the tension. Some teens with anxiety are acutely self-conscious and embarrassed by their symptoms, which may lead to shame and suicidal thoughts or behaviors.

Substance Use

Although a few children and many adolescents experiment with drugs and alcohol, for some teens substance use goes beyond more typical experimentation and can become an addiction as well as a way of attempting to cope with problems. More extreme substance use, especially when the teen also has a psychiatric disorder, is especially concerning as a risk factor for suicide. Drugs and alcohol lower inhibitions, impair the ability to think clearly and make good choices, and increase the likelihood that someone will act impulsively. Thus, many suicide attempts are made when the person is intoxicated. In addition, having a substance problem is a significant stressor in itself and can cause teens to feel they have even less control over their lives and futures.

Trauma and Posttraumatic Stress Disorder

Children and adolescents who have been physically or sexually abused, or who have witnessed significant domestic violence or other violent events, are coping with much more stress than the average child. This puts them at greater risk for mental health issues, behavioral problems, and suicide. Their traumatic experiences may cause them to feel unable to trust others or that the world is an inherently unsafe and unreliable place. They may feel intense shame, blame themselves for the traumatic event, or feel so besieged by traumatic memories that they feel self-harm or suicide is the only way to cope. A subset of children who have been exposed to traumatic events have symptoms that meet criteria for PTSD and/or other psychiatric disorders, which further increases their risk for self-harm.

Psychosis

Psychosis is a thought disorder and occurs when someone's ability to identify reality is impaired. It is very rare in children and uncommon in adolescents, but it can occur secondary to other psychiatric diagnoses including depression, bipolar disorder, and schizophrenia. Psychotic symptoms include perceptual disturbances such as auditory and visual hallucinations as well as delusional thinking. Other more subtle signs that someone might be psychotic include becoming more isolative, poor attention to personal hygiene, withdrawal from normal activities, and statements or communication that does not make sense. Certain psychotic symptoms are particularly dangerous. Some youths experience auditory hallucinations in which "the voices told me to cut" or "the voices told me to kill myself," and these youths are at very high risk for suicide and self-harm. Other youths have delusions that are very frightening to them, such as that they are evil or cursed, and may lead to suicidal thoughts or behaviors. Even if these symptoms are treated, adolescents newly diagnosed with a psychotic disorder, such as schizophrenia, are at increased risk for suicide as they struggle to come to terms with their new diagnosis and its ramifications for their future.

Attention-Deficit/Hyperactivity Disorder

Although suicidality and self-injurious behaviors are not typical in children diagnosed with attention-deficit/hyperactivity disorder (ADHD), these children are often impulsive and may not think clearly about the consequences of their actions before acting. This can raise the risk that they will do something to harm themselves in the midst of a conflict, during a stressful moment, or when experiencing a strong emotion without fully considering the possible outcomes or being able to think rationally about alternative ways of coping. In addition, children with ADHD often have difficulty regulating their emotions and so may be less able to tolerate a stressful situation and respond appropriately.

Autism Spectrum Disorder

Many youths with autism spectrum disorder are prone to rigid, black-and-white thinking, impulsive behavior, and difficulty managing frustration. They can also often be targets of teasing or bullying by peers or be socially isolated because they seem "odd" to peers. This can put them at increased risk of suicide when faced with acute stress.

Identifying Immediate Triggers

When a child or teen makes a suicidal statement or engages in self-harm, detailed information should be gathered to fully understand the **context** in which the statement or behavior occurred. This can be done through a detailed discussion with the child or a "chain analysis" where the events, **immediate stressors,** thoughts, and feelings of the child leading up to and immediately following the event are described and recorded (Table 3–2). In the case of self-injury such as cutting, the child should be asked about the period leading up to the cutting, aspects of which could include more general stressors over the past several weeks, events earlier that day, specific thoughts or feelings, any attempts to cope in other ways, the decision or impulse to cut, where and when the child cut, what instrument he used to cut, how he obtained it, how he cut, and what he thought, felt, and did afterwards, as well as the reaction of anyone else that became aware of the cutting. This provides an opportunity for a discussion about where in the chain of events the child or teen could have done something differently or where he could have obtained support from others. The same approach can be used to evaluate any triggers which precipitated a suicidal statement or behavior.

Risk Assessment

Children or teens who are considering suicide or who are injuring themselves often show some **warning signs,** even if they cannot directly ask for help. Warning signs to watch out for include becoming more withdrawn, isolative, irritable, anxious, or unmotivated; not taking care of personal hygiene, schoolwork, or other important activities; experiencing changes in eating or sleeping; using drugs or alcohol; and expressing hopelessness about the future, or feelings of low self-esteem, guilt, or worthlessness. Children who start talking about death or dying, who give away their belongings, or who write a suicide note are at very high risk.

It is also important to consider the **context** or **environment.** A child who is socially isolated, or who is struggling with a recent rejection or loss such as death, divorce, or a breakup, is at much greater risk. Often, when asked directly and in a quiet, safe and private place, children and teens will be honest about suicidal thoughts and self-harm.

Onsite Stabilization

There is a common misconception that talking about suicide might "put the idea in their head" and cause children to make a suicide attempt. This is not the case. In fact, open communication about suicide in a calm and nonjudgmental manner sends the message to teens that adults care about them, are able to handle these issues, and know how to help. Having had these discussions makes it more likely that a child or teen in trouble will reach out for help from a parent, teacher, guidance counselor, or coach.

TABLE 3–2. Risk factors and immediate triggers for suicide and self-injury

Environmental factors	Prior suicide by a peer or family member
	Domestic violence
	Physical abuse or neglect
	Bullying or cyberbullying
	Social isolation
	Family stress
Child factors	Depression
	Impulsivity
	Previous self-harm or suicide attempts
	Hopelessness
	Ideas about death as a relief from suffering
	Sleep problems
	History of abuse or trauma
	Substance use
	Difficulties with communication or problem solving
	Sexual minority youths
Psychiatric illness	Mood disorders (depressive disorders, bipolar disorder)
	Substance use
	Trauma and posttraumatic stress disorder
	Psychosis
	Autism spectrum disorder
	Attention-deficit/hyperactivity disorder
	Anxiety disorders
	Obsessive-compulsive disorder
Immediate triggers	Feeling of shame or rejection
	Teasing by peers
	Breakup or loss
	Reminders of traumatic experiences or abuse
	Family conflict

Similarly, thoughtful discussion regarding self-injury can have an important impact for at-risk children and teens.

If a teacher, parent, coach, or pediatrician discovers that a child has been feeling suicidal or has been engaging in self-harm, onsite stabilization in the moment of crisis should include providing the child with support and the message that she is important and cared about. Children who have indicated that they are thinking about suicide, or who have intentionally harmed themselves, should be provided with a calm, private place to talk about how they are feeling, and to discuss any incidents that led them to make a suicidal statement or to self-harm while the adults involved determine next steps. The child should not be left alone at any point if there is suspicion that she is or has recently been suicidal.

Removing access to potential means for suicide or for self-harm is important if you have identified a child at risk. This is particularly important when it comes to firearms, but other dangerous items, including medications, pesticides, toxic household substances, and knives and other sharp objects, should also be removed and locked in a place that children and teens cannot access. Parents should be educated about making these changes to the home environment if their child or adolescent is at risk for suicide or self-injurious behaviors.

Catch the Warning Signs

School personnel, pediatricians, religious leaders, youth workers, coaches, and parents know children best and are in the best position to pick up on the warning signs that something is wrong. Warning signs, as discussed earlier, include physical evidence of cutting or burning; talking about death or dying; drug or alcohol use; hopelessness about the future; recent loss; changes in personality or motivation; social withdrawal; loss of interest in activities; poor sleep, eating, hygiene, or concentration; changes in school performance; bizarre or erratic behavior; and feelings of low self-esteem, guilt, or worthlessness.

Listen and Empathize

If a child has been cutting herself or engaging in self-injury, ask about it without judgment to understand the child's perspective. It can be painful for an adult to discover that a child they care about has been hurting herself, but try to stay calm and avoid strong emotions, as often the child has been hiding the self-harm for fear of upsetting others. Ask the child when and how she hurt herself, what her intention was at the time with particular attention to whether she harmed herself with suicidal intent or for other reasons, any factors or stressors that led up to the self-injury, what she used to hurt herself, how she felt after, and whether she was having thoughts of doing it again. Any injury should be visually inspected to determine if the child requires medical attention such as stitches. This information can be used to determine what level of follow-up care is appropriate, including school-based counseling, potentially notifying parents, referral for outpatient therapy, or referral to the emergency room (ER).

Collaborate to Find Solutions

The child should be part of the discussion about next steps or follow-up after the crisis. Often the child will ask that things be kept secret, and it is important to be honest with the child about who will be notified and why. If a parent will be informed, the child should be told this and given an opportunity to tell the parent herself or to be present when this happens. The need to ensure the child's safety should be emphasized as the first priority and rationale for informing others.

Determining whether to tell a parent that a child has intentionally injured herself can be a difficult decision. In most cases it will be important that the parent or caregiver responsible for the child understand that this has occurred so that they can be part of preventing future self-injury and in addressing whatever underlying issues contributed to this behavior. Caregivers will often need to remove dangerous objects from the home following an incident of self-injury and will also often need to seek treatment for their child. In rare cases, such as when a child scratches herself very superficially for the first time, the clinician may decide to address this with the child directly without immediately informing a parent; however, this decision should be carefully considered, because most often self-injury is a sign children will need increased support and monitoring, including at home.

When a child at school or other program is found to be suicidal, parents should be notified immediately and should come to pick up the child and talk with the staff about what the child has said. If the parent is safely able to bring the child to a mental health professional (preferably one who already knows the child) for immediate evaluation, this should be done the same day. If the parent is not able to arrange to have the child seen the same day, the child should be taken to the hospital for evaluation in the ER. If the child is too aggressive, disorganized, angry, or unpredictable for a parent to safely bring her to the hospital, emergency medical services should be called and the child should be escorted to the hospital via ambulance, again with a parent accompanying her. If a parent or caregiver is unavailable, another trusted adult should accompany the child. If the child has taken an overdose or has cut herself deeply, 911 should be called and the child should be taken to the ER immediately for both medical and psychiatric evaluation.

Learning From the Crisis

Once the immediate crisis has ended and the child is calm, sit down with the child to revisit the incident. This is an opportunity to review what took place, identify triggers and stressors, and find alternative ways of coping in the future. The child can be asked where in the process she and others could have acted differently and what would have been helpful. This can help the child to identify coping strategies she can use in the future, and also what to do if she feels overwhelmed and needs to ask for help. Help the child to develop a safety plan she can use should suicidal thoughts or urges to self-harm return. A safety plan should include the names of those whom the child will reach out to for help both during the day and at night, the contact information for those individuals, and emergency procedures to be used if they are unreachable, such as calling 911 or going to an ER.

Family and community supports are key in helping at-risk kids, and supportive and engaging school programming and extracurricular activities can also be helpful to prevent future suicide or self-harm. Kids who feel connected to their schools and communities and who are busy and connected to positive after-school activities are less vulnerable to the issues and stressors that contribute to depression, risk-taking, self-injury, and suicidality.

When to Get Help

Youths who are cutting themselves, expressing hopeless feelings, or sharing suicidal thoughts should always be referred for mental health treatment. Dialectical behavior therapy is a specific type of therapy that is especially effective in helping adolescents with persistent suicidality or self-injurious behavior (Groves et al. 2012) and should be considered when referring youths for treatment when available. Self-injurious behavior may not always require immediate psychiatric assessment in an ER, but as it is often reflective of underlying depression, substance use, or other psychological stressors, youths who self-harm should be connected to an experienced therapist or psychiatrist. Suicidal statements or attempts should always be evaluated by trained mental health professionals. If a child has expressed suicidal thoughts, has made a suicide attempt, or has been identified as engaging in high-risk self-injury, he should be immediately evaluated by a psychiatrist or psychologist. If the child is already working with such a clinician, the child can be taken to see that clinician the same day. If the child in not already in treatment, he should be brought to the local ER for evaluation. Evaluation in the ER will involve an interview with the child and caregivers as well as communication with others who know the child well. Once in the ER, the child will often minimize or deny having made suicidal statements or engaged in self-harm, because he is embarrassed, frightened, or worried about upsetting his parents. Emergency doctors depend strongly on the school staff, therapists, and others who know the child well to understand what has really been going on and assess the level of risk. It is immensely helpful to the mental health team evaluating the child if school personnel who are sending the child for evaluation send a letter detailing the reason the child is being sent, a description of what took place, any observed changes in the child's behavior, and what concerns they have about the child's functioning or safety.

References

Anderson R, Smith BL: Deaths: leading causes for 2002. Natl Vital Stat Rep 53(17):1–89, 2005

Centers for Disease Control and Prevention, National Center for Injury Prevention and Control: Suicide prevention: youth suicide, 2007. Available at: http://www.cdc.gov/violenceprevention/pub/youth_suicide.html. Accessed June 11, 2014.

Centers for Disease Control and Prevention. Youth risk behavior surveillance–United States, 2011. MMWR Surveill Summ 61(4), June 8, 2012. Available from www.cdc.gov/mmwr/pdf/ss/ss6104.pdf. Accessed June 11, 2014.

Crosby AE, Ortega L, Melanson C: Self-Directed Violence Surveillance: Uniform Definitions and Recommended Data Elements, Version 1.0. Atlanta, GA, Centers for Disease Control and Prevention, National Center for Injury Prevention and Control, 2011

Fleischmann A, Bertolote JM, Belfer M, Beautrais A: Completed suicide and psychiatric diagnoses in young people: a critical examination of the evidence. Am J Orthopsychiatry 75(4):676–683, 2005

Groves S, Backer H, van den Bosch W, Miller A: Review: dialectical behaviour therapy with adolescents. Child and Adolescent Mental Health 17(2):65–75, 2012

Guan K, Fox KR, Prinstein MJ: Nonsuicidal self-injury as a time-invariant predictor of adolescent suicide ideation and attempts in a diverse community sample. J Consult Clin Psychol 80(5):842–849, 2012

Liu R, Mustanski B: Suicidal ideation and self-harm in lesbian, gay, bisexual, and transgender youth. Am J Prevent Med 42(3):221–228, 2012

Nock M, Green J, Hwang I, et al: Prevalence, correlates, and treatment of lifetime suicidal behavior among adolescents: results from the National Comorbidity Survey Replication Adolescent Supplement. JAMA Psychiatry 70(3)300–310, 2013

Posner K, Brown GK, Stanley B, et al: The Columbia-Suicide Severity Rating Scale: initial validity and internal consistency findings from three multisite studies with adolescents and adults. Am J Psychiatry 168:1266–1277, 2011

Saewyc E, Chen W: To what extent can adolescent suicide attempts be attributed to violence exposure? A population-based study from Western Canada. Can J Commun Ment Health 32(1):79–94, 2013

Wolitzky-Taylor KB, Ruggiero KJ, McCart MR, et al: Has adolescent suicidality decreased in the United States? Data from two national samples of adolescents interviewed in 1995 and 2005. J Clin Child Adolesc Psychol 39(1):64–76, 2010

Consider Risk Factors
1. Talking about dying
2. Recent loss, including death, divorce, or a breakup
3. Change in personality, including becoming more withdrawn, isolative, irritable, anxious, or unmotivated
4. Changes in behavior, including poor concentration, deteriorating school performance, poor hygiene, or lack of energy
5. Changes in appetite or eating, changes in sleep
6. Drug or alcohol use
7. Aggressive or erratic behavior
8. Loss of interest in activities and/or time with friends
9. Feelings of low self-esteem, guilt, or worthlessness
10. Hopelessness about the future or about the possibility that things will improve
11. Bizarre or disorganized behavior

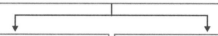

De-escalation	**Refer to the Emergency Room if:**
1. Find a private space for the child to talk.	1. The child reports suicidal thoughts.
2. Provide support and encouragement.	2. The child has cut or burned or intentionally injured herself in the recent past.
3. Listen to what the child has to say.	3. The child appears significantly depressed or hopeless and cannot identify ways of coping.
4. Ask about what is wrong, how the child feels, and what might help.	4. The adult involved feels unsure in any way that the child will be safe.
5. Ask whether the child has thought about wanting to die or hurting herself.	
6. Ask whether the child has acted on thoughts of hurting herself.	

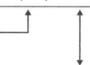

Learn From the Crisis and Refer for Outpatient Treatment if:
1. The child has not reported any suicidal thoughts and not hurt herself.
2. The child appears to be depressed or anxious or using substances.
3. There has been trauma exposure, loss, or a major transition in the child's life.
4. The child seems to be dealing with an increase in stressors.

Managing a suicidal child in crisis.

CHAPTER 4

Tantrums and Behavioral Outbursts

M. Cevdet Tosyali, M.D.

Tantrums, as anyone who has ever interacted with a young child knows, are highly disruptive displays of negative emotion that begin early in childhood (with 50% of children having tantrums before their first birthday). They are almost universal–by 36 months almost all children will have developed tantrums and temper outbursts (breath-holding spells are considered by many to also fall into this category). But their universality does not make tantrums any easier to deal with. They are a huge source of strain on parents and teachers and disrupt family outings, doctor's appointments, supermarket visits, classrooms, sleep schedules, and other routines.

The universality of tantrums can make it difficult to tell where normal development ends and psychopathology begins. Temper dysregulation is a component of many mental disorders, but the vast majority of temper tantrums are not reflective of major mental illness. Still, tantrums and outbursts remain the most common cause for mental health clinic referrals and also for inpatient psychiatric hospitalizations in children and adolescents (Carlson et al. 2009).

In evaluating and responding to tantrums, then, it is crucial not to over-pathologize normal developmental events, yet simultaneously important to recognize when tantrums are beyond what is normal for a child's age and cognitive level. By doing so we can identify and help those children who are lagging behind in cognitive, language, or problem-solving skills, and also recognize which children are in the early stages of disruptive behavior disorders, depression, or other mental health problems (Burke et al. 2010; Nock et al. 2007; Stringaris and Goodman 2009; Stringaris et al. 2010; Wakschlag et al. 2014).

Case Presentation

Joseph, a normally energetic pre-K student, is brought into the counselor's office by Tina, his new student teacher. Today, Joseph seems not himself—he is quiet, pouty, and decisively unresponsive to Tina as she tries to console him with a lively voice and wavy arms. Tina reports that Joseph, one of the wonderful students in Mrs. G's pre-K class, has seemed a bit sad lately. At times he is his usual energetic self, but at other times he seems slowed down, lagging behind, and having trouble moving from one activity to the next. For example, when asked to leave the toy corner yesterday, he began to have a tantrum, scream, knock over some books, then cry and roll around on the rug for 5–10 minutes. Tina tried various positive reinforcement strategies, including showing him nice books he might like so he could choose the book they would all read, making funny faces to make him laugh, and telling him he should see the bright side and be positive because he would be able to return to play after reading and then arts and crafts. She even tried being stern and telling him he really had to join the rest of the class "or else," but that didn't work either. Today, instead of a few books, he knocked down a whole bookshelf, which was not big, and it was definitely by mistake, but it did scrape Tina's arm on the way down. It was just a small scrape, but Mrs. G said Joseph's mother should be called and he should go to the emergency room (ER) for an evaluation because he was a danger to himself or others.

Understanding the Crisis

Tantrums in a preschooler like Joseph are, as noted earlier, extremely common. They follow a typical pattern over a child's early life. Infants and very young children experience distress (hunger, fatigue, anger, frustration) without having either the ability to put words to their experience or the cognitive or physical skill to solve the problem that is producing the distress. As children progress through toddlerhood, they learn to differentiate these feelings to some degree, and tantrums begin to take a certain standard form (Wakschlag et al. 2012). They begin with anger, which is high amplitude and short lived, usually peaking within 1 minute, and continue with distress, which is low amplitude and of longer duration (Potegal et al. 1996, 2009; Qiu et al. 2009). As kids get older and become more able to express their feelings and wants verbally, learn to soothe themselves, and realize that adults will not give in even if they have a tantrum, these behaviors decline, and most children will no longer exhibit tantrums by school age.

If tantrums persist past kindergarten, this is reason for concern. Tantrums occurring daily, even in young children, or regularly lasting longer than 10 minutes should also be a red flag that this is outside of the norm (Belden et al. 2008; Goodenough 1975; Wakschlag et al. 2012). Tantrums that occur with parents are extremely common, whereas frequent tantrums at school or with other adults such as grandparents are more unusual, occurring in only one-third of children. For most children, tantrums are fairly predictable, occurring in repetitive ways such as in the grocery store checkout line or when the child is asked to stop playing and come to dinner. If the tantrums are unpredictable, without any pattern, this should raise concern. Another potential red flag is if a child has "grown out" of tantrums and then the tantrums reemerge or become more frequent or severe.

Individual tantrum behaviors, such as cursing, hitting, head banging, or breaking things, are actually not an indicator of mental illness or deeper problems. This is particularly true in older children or adolescents whose temper outbursts routinely involve foul language, property destruction, or even verbal threats, even though the outbursts are identical to a toddler's temper tantrum in function and origins (Potegal et al. 2009). The one exception to this rule is self-harm behaviors (e.g., cutting or slapping oneself), which should raise concern for depression.

To summarize, the following are major red flags that suggest when tantrums are beyond what is developmentally normal (Potegal and Davidson 2003):

- Aggression against caregivers
- Intentional self-injury during a tantrum
- Frequent tantrums, with 10–20 tantrums on separate days at home in a 30-day period, or more than 5 tantrums a day at home or school or outside
- Extended duration of tantrums, with tantrums lasting 25 minutes on average
- Inability to self-soothe

Identifying Kids at Risk for Tantrums and Behavioral Outbursts

When tantrums increase in frequency or severity or reemerge after a child has "grown out" of such behaviors, oftentimes the culprit in these cases is **changes in the child's health or in the environment.** Many children are very sensitive to **sleep deprivation, hunger,** or **social environment.** Changes in bedtime or daytime routine, interruptions in sleep (e.g., due to a new baby brother who cries at night, or nightmares after a scary event or even a scary movie) can have a direct effect on temper. Minor **physical discomforts,** such as a stomachache or earache, can lead to tantrums (either directly, because the child is frustrated by the pain, or indirectly if the child is more irritable and less able to manage other frustrations or stress). More significant **medical problems** can also increase temper problems in children and adolescents, with acute or chronic effects. Thyroid illness is particularly important, because it is closely linked to mood an anxiety disorders. For other medical illnesses, the treatment itself can lead to temper problems; asthma medication and steroids are just two categories of treatment that at times can have such effects. Finally, **environmental changes** must be considered. Seemingly simple changes such as a sibling's absence from home due to beginning school or a change in caregivers or in routine, and obviously important factors such as a change in school or residence, parental absence or separation, illness or death in the family, financial difficulty, parental job loss, and parental discord, may all lead to an increase in outbursts.

Children with **cognitive limitations, learning disabilities,** or **language disorders** are at increased risk for tantrums as well. When these children are upset, it is difficult for them to express their feelings and needs verbally. They also often have difficulty solving problems, because this requires verbal and social skills. When frustration mounts and these children are unable to find a solution, they will often have a tantrum and may begin hitting, kicking, or throwing things. We often tell kids during a tantrum to "use your words," but children with cognitive or language disabilities will not be able to do so without specific therapy and supports to teach them these skills. Even children who are not formally diagnosed with a learning disability but who are less articulate or less socially adept than their peers can be vulnerable to this. And if parents, teachers, or others then "give in" and let the child have what he wants to calm him, this can reinforce for the child that having a tantrum is a way to get his needs met.

Family factors can also make a child more vulnerable to tantrums. In families where there are many children, where parents are stressed and stretched, or where a single parent is overwhelmed with juggling work and child care, a child may have more tantrums in a desperate attempt to get the parent's attention. If there is conflict in the home, either physical violence or the more typical yelling and arguing, this may teach a child that yelling and throwing things is a way to get what she wants. If there are multiple caregivers taking care of the child, particularly if they have different rules or routines or if there is conflict between them, the child is more likely to get confused and frustrated and then have a tantrum, or to try to use tantrums to get her way. Conflict in the home or a parent being very stressed and strained can also make the child anxious. An anxious child will be more on edge and vulnerable to tantrums and outbursts; this is even more true if the parent is depressed (including postpartum depression), severely anxious, or otherwise ill. In these cases, treating the parent's illness will often eliminate the tantrums even without any treatment for the child or any parenting intervention (Wickramaratne et al. 2011). Finally, if the child does not have a father or father figure in the home, this can increase tantrums as well. Children (particularly boys with attention or behavioral problems) often respond better to their father's limit setting and discipline than to their mother's.

Differential Diagnosis

When temper tantrums fall outside the norm in the ways described earlier, they may be a sign of mental illness. And when children with mental illness have tantrums, these can be important moments to identify unresolved symptoms or difficulties. Your observations of the tantrum and the events leading up to it will be incredibly useful to the clinician evaluating the child to ensure the right diagnosis and treatment are given.

Oppositional Defiant Disorder and Conduct Disorder

Nine out of 10 children who are referred to a psychiatrist for tantrums have a presentation that meets criteria for oppositional defiant disorder (ODD) (Kochanska et al. 2001). Children with ODD—which affects about 5% of the population—are persistently angry, irritable, argumentative, defiant, and even vindictive. Some amount of defiance is present in all young children; kids will refuse to do something or attempt to negotiate with the parent ("Five more minutes! Let me finish this level!") but are responsive when the parent holds firm or repeats the instruction. Children with ODD have more defiant refusal, often with more anger or distress, and do not back down. Children with ODD are headstrong, rigid, and argumentative with parents and teachers, and may be less mindful of others' emotions or the effects of their behavior on others. They are often irritable and easily frustrated, and they are vulnerable to tantrums because of the frequent conflict that occurs as a result of their argumentativeness and also because they are less able to handle frustration than their peers and siblings who do not have ODD. Children with ODD often have other mental illnesses as well, including attention-deficit/hyperactivity disorder (ADHD), depression, learning disabilities, and anxiety disorders. When a child with ODD has a tantrum, it is important to look at what set it off–for example, being told no, feelings of frustration, or conflict with peers–so that in treatment you can teach the child ways to manage that in the future.

A small number of children with ODD go on to develop conduct disorder, which includes behaviors such as property destruction, theft, deceit, and severe aggression. Children who are exposed to physical abuse or physical discipline may be more likely to become aggressive; they may also have different character traits like low fear, little attention to others' emotions or social cues, and little emotional upset when being punished. These children are more likely to attribute hostility to others, so that if a peer bumps into them accidentally in the hallway, they are more likely to perceive a threat and then perhaps pitch a fit. Exposure to a warm and nurturing caregiver may protect children from developing conduct disorder over time, so early identification is important.

Attention-Deficit/Hyperactivity Disorder

Although attention problems, hyperactivity, and impulsivity are the core symptoms of ADHD, emotion dysregulation is present in a majority of children with ADHD. Tantrums and outbursts bring many children with ADHD to treatment, and among children with tantrums and outbursts referred for evaluation, ADHD is second only to ODD in frequency of diagnosis, with rates above 70% (Roy et al. 2013). Temper dysregulation in ADHD often improves with appropriate ADHD treatment with stimulant medications, but behavioral therapies can also be useful, particularly for children with ADHD and ODD (Sonuga-Barke et al. 2013). Tantrums and temper outbursts in children with ADHD and ODD may be slightly different from those in children with ADHD only. Children with ODD are more likely to mope or sulk throughout the day after an outburst, whereas children with ADHD alone tend to return to their normal happy, hyperactive selves quickly after a tantrum. Children with ADHD are also at high risk for having comorbid learning disabilities.

Autism Spectrum Disorder

From nearly 1.5% (Developmental Disabilities Monitoring Network Surveillance Year 2010 Principal Investigators 2014) to more than 2% (Kim et al. 2014) of the population have autism spectrum disorder, with symptoms of marked deficiency in social communication usually apparent by age 2 years, though sometimes the diagnosis is not made until much later. Tantrums and outbursts are more prevalent in children with autism spectrum disorder than they are in typically developing children (Tureck et al. 2014). Unlike in typically developing children or even children with intellectual disability, outbursts in children with autism may begin without any discernible reason, may vary greatly in duration and severity, and may cease as suddenly as they began. Autistic children's tantrums often involve stereotyped, repetitive behaviors (e.g., flapping or head banging) and minor aggression (e.g., pinching or pulling hair). Tantrums in children with autism are often communications of distress or discomfort (including overstimulation by sound, light, or physical sensations such as clothing textures), or a means of escaping from an upsetting stimulus. Children with autism may be more prone to tantrums because of rigidity and difficulty with transitions, because they are sensitive to noise and light, and because they lack the social skills to solve problems or ask effectively for what they want or need. Understanding the triggers for tantrums in children with autism can be difficult because, with the language deficits often present in autism, the child may be unable to tell you what upset him or what he wants. A careful behavioral analysis can be helpful to identify triggers for tantrums as well as particular times or places where the child is vulnerable to tantrums (e.g., during a transition from one classroom to another, in the grocery store or restaurant, at bathtime). Once the triggers and vulnerability points are identified, a behavior plan can be put into place to help the child manage these situations (and it may be recommended that the child avoid certain places, like the grocery store, altogether).

Autism is frequently comorbid with ADHD, and children with autism and ADHD combined are more likely to have tantrums than children with either autism or ADHD alone (Goldin et al. 2013). Temper outbursts in children with autism and ADHD are more severe, more frequent, and more impairing than in children with either autism or ADHD alone, and are often more difficult to treat.

Learning Disabilities and Intellectual Disability

Children with unrecognized learning disabilities may be more likely to have tantrums in the classroom because they are frustrated or embarrassed that they are not keeping up with the class, or because they are teased by peers for their difficulties. Intellectual disability also increases risk for tantrums and outbursts, though this varies greatly among individuals depending on the degree of disability, temperament, and the presence of comorbid psychiatric problems such as autism, ADHD, ODD, or particular learning disabilities. There are also a number of genetic syndromes that lead to intellectual disability and that also have very high rates of outbursts, which can be prolonged, can contain aggression against self and others, and may prove difficult to treat. Syndromes with increased outbursts include cri du chat, Smith-Magenis, Prader-Willi, Angelman, Cornelia de Lange, and fragile X syndromes.

Tourette's Disorder

Tourette's disorder (often abbreviated "TS" for Tourette's syndrome) is a neuropsychiatric disorder involving multiple motor and vocal tics. Children with Tourette's disorder can also have tantrums, rages, explosive outbursts, and rarely (in about 15% of kids) compulsive swearing, called *coprolalia*. These rages and outbursts are present mostly in kids who have Tourette's disorder together with other psychiatric disorders such as obsessive-compulsive disorder (OCD), ADHD, ODD, and autism spectrum disorder.

Temper tantrums and rages in individuals with Tourette's disorder seem to be mostly associated with ADHD, though there are cases in which ADHD symptoms are minimal and yet rages are significant. Outbursts in individuals with Tourette's disorder are usually high-anger events that can begin instantaneously but also tend to dissipate quickly. They are very difficult to treat with psychotherapeutic interventions, although psychopharmacological treatment of children with comorbid diagnoses such as ADHD and OCD can reduce the frequency and severity of tantrums (Alsobrook and Pauls 2002; Cheung et al. 2007).

Children with Tourette's disorder usually first develop motor tics around age 5–7 years, although onset of tics can occur as early as age 2 years or as late as age 20 years. In many children with tics, ADHD will be the first obvious concern, though retrospective review often indicates symptoms of OCD in early childhood. Tics and later noticeable OCD will then follow. Tics may be simple, such as blinking or twitching of the nose, head, or trunk, or complex, such as squatting or jumping. Simple vocalizations then develop; sniffing, snorting, grunting, throat clearing, and coughing are common, though complex vocal tics, such as those consisting of strings of words and animal noises, also occur. Tic severity usually increases until roughly 12 years of age, after which decline is common.

Bipolar Disorder, Disruptive Mood Dysregulation Disorder, and Depression

Tantrums and temper outbursts can occur in the context of mood disorders as well. Many children with frequent irritability and tantrums are diagnosed as having bipolar disorder, but an accurate bipolar disorder diagnosis requires that irritability occur only in distinct, well-demarcated episodes in which the child is also having other symptoms, including decreased need for sleep, racing thoughts, disorganized thinking, fast and pressured speech, unusual impulsivity, grandiosity, and psychomotor agitation, all of which do not occur when the adolescent is not having a mood episode. Children who are always silly, impulsive, distractible, or energetic and then have frequent tantrums are more likely to have ADHD than bipolar disorder. Bipolar disorder in childhood is quite rare, and most children with tantrums—even very severe tantrums—do not have bipolar disorder.

A newer diagnosis, disruptive mood dysregulation disorder (DMDD), does a better job of describing children with chronic irritability and frequent tantrums. Chronic, severe irritability, occurring most days and observable by others, is its core feature. Temper outbursts are required as a manifestation of this irritability, and diagnosis requires severe, recurrent (i.e., three or more times a week) temper outbursts that are inconsistent with developmental level. These symptoms must exist in at least two settings and be present for a minimum of 12 months without any interruption lasting 3 months or longer (American Psychiatric Association 2013). DMDD appears to be a form of irritable depression and is associated with an increased risk for depression (not bipolar disorder) in adolescence and adulthood (Baroni et al. 2009; Stringaris et al. 2010).

It is also important to consider depression when children and adolescents are referred for tantrums. One-third of children referred for evaluation of tantrums and outbursts have depression, often along with ODD. Most children with depression do not have severe tantrums, but depression combined with ODD can lead to longer and more severe tantrums. Also important, self-harming behaviors during tantrums, which are rare in the absence of autism or intellectual disability, seem to appear only in depressed children (Belden et al. 2008).

Anxiety Disorders, Obsessive-Compulsive Disorder, and Posttraumatic Stress Disorder

Anxiety disorders, as well as OCD and posttraumatic stress disorder (PTSD), are diagnosed in up to 50% of children with tantrums and outbursts, and they have high rates of a family history of anxiety disorders (Roy et al. 2013). Often the tantrums are related to spikes of anxiety or attempts to escape something that is anxiety provoking. For example, if a child with separation anxiety is asked to separate from dad when she gets to preschool, she may throw a tantrum both as a manifestation of her severe anxiety, and perhaps to encourage dad to stick around (which would decrease her anxiety).

Similarly, a child with OCD who is prevented from engaging in his compulsive checking or washing might have a tantrum or outburst because his anxiety becomes unbearable. OCD may also coexist with ADHD and at times with Tourette's disorder, which could account for even greater tantrum and outburst behavior. Forced separation in a child with separation anxiety may lead to disruptive behavior and outbursts. PTSD may be associated outbursts related to triggers or trauma reminders that lead to intense reexperiencing of the traumatic event; reexperiencing may manifest with agitation and aggression as the child feels all the fear and anxiety of the initial trauma. All of these situations are capable of being repeated daily in susceptible children. Diagnosis of separation anxiety may be straightforward, but OCD and PTSD may remain hidden in children.

Identifying Immediate Triggers

When one of the psychiatric disorders described in the preceding section is present, the child may be vulnerable to tantrums, but mental illness is unlikely to directly cause tantrums without some other trigger or provoking event (Table 4–1). Often the child will have difficulty saying what has set him or her off, but trying to understand the experience from the child's perspective can be helpful. For example, in our case example, is Joseph more vulnerable to tantrums because his dad has been traveling and his mom has been stressed, and Joseph is feeling more sad or on edge as a result? Does he have difficulty with transitions because he has undiagnosed autism such that the trigger of shifting from playtime to circle time keeps setting him off? Or does he have difficulty with circle time because he has undiagnosed ADHD and has difficulty sitting still and gets frustrated and then has a tantrum? Have other kids been teasing him, and has his language disability or social skills deficit made it hard for him to ask the teacher for help? Or is it something as simple as being hungry, having an earache, or needing to use the bathroom and he just does not know how to express what he needs?

It is also important to pay attention to changes in the child's behavior and mood. If a child who never had tantrums before is now having them regularly, something may have changed at home, or it may be she is sick (medically or psychiatrically), or she may be having trouble keeping up with the increasing demands of school (either academically or socially). Watching for signs of depression or anxiety is key, because these are often missed. Depressed or anxious children get frustrated and upset more easily and might have a tantrum because of simple conflicts or problems, such as forgetting their homework at home or not understanding their assignments. It is crucial to identify the immediate triggers and try to address them both to de-escalate the situation and to prevent future tantrums.

TABLE 4–1. Risk factors and immediate triggers for tantrums

Environmental factors	Family stress
	Depressed, anxious, or medically ill parent
	Domestic violence at home
	Physical discipline at home
	Neglect (if the child is hungry or not sleeping well)
	Chaotic home or multiple caregivers
Child factors	Unrecognized learning disability or social skills deficits
	Intellectual disability
	Medical illness
	Hunger, fatigue, or physical discomfort
Psychiatric illness	Autism spectrum disorder
	Attention-deficit/hyperactivity disorder
	Oppositional defiant disorder or conduct disorder
	Anxiety disorders, including separation anxiety
	Obsessive-compulsive disorder
	Posttraumatic stress disorder
	Mood disorders (depression, bipolar disorder, disruptive mood dysregulation disorder)
Immediate triggers	Teasing by peers
	Classwork that is too difficult
	Hunger or pain
	Stress or environmental changes at home
	Overstimulation (particularly for kids with autism)

Risk Assessment

As noted earlier, most tantrums are benign, mild, and normative. But tantrums can become severe and dangerous, especially if the child starts throwing objects at others or harming himself by banging his body or head on the floor. Keeping the child safe during the tantrum is our number one priority. As was discussed in previous chapters, make sure that the **environment** is safe–that the child is well observed, not left alone in the room, and prevented from accessing sharp objects or any object that could be thrown and harm others. If someone else in the room is setting the child off, either directly or indirectly (sometimes more attention serves to increase the tantrum behavior, even if that was not the trigger for the tantrum), try to remove those additional people, and make sure the child is with someone he feels safe with and close to. Second, consider the child's **history.** If a child has a history of intense, lengthy, and dangerous tantrums, you will manage this child's case differently than if the child is known to have brief outbursts but recover quickly. Also, consider what has helped or not helped in the past. Finally, consider the child's **current behavior** and level of agitation. If the child is hurting himself (either on purpose or accidentally), take whatever steps are needed to keep him safe. If the child is at risk for hurting someone else, remove the others or move the child to a safe place while you work with your team to figure out your next steps.

Onsite Stabilization

As most tantrums are not reflective of mental illness or acute or severe problems, they will not require calling 911 or a trip to the ER, which leaves you with the task of de-escalating the tantrum onsite. Many tantrums can be stopped before they become a crisis. Even when the tantrum is so severe, prolonged, or violent that an emergency psychiatric evaluation is indicated, you will need to attempt to contain and de-escalate the child before emergency medical services personnel arrive, to ensure the safety of the child and others around him.

Catch the Warning Signs

The best way to avoid a tantrum becoming severe or dangerous is to prevent it entirely. Children do not go from 0 to 60 immediately; there is a ramp-up period that is the first point for potential intervention. The first sign is often a subtle change in emotion, moving toward the initial anger phase of the tantrum. Intervening at this point requires speed, because the child's affect can switch abruptly; the window of opportunity is very narrow, closing quickly.

One potential way to avert a tantrum is to give the child whatever it was that he wanted or needed in the first place. This may seem foolish and counterproductive, but it is not. The most detrimental response is to wait until the child has had a major meltdown and then give him the thing he wanted, as the child then learns that he can get what he wants through having a tantrum, and the tantrum is reinforced as a useful strategy for attaining goals. If you suspect that you will end up "caving in" to the child's request in the end if he has a tantrum, giving the desired thing in advance can avoid both the outburst and the reinforcement of outbursts as a coping strategy. Ask yourself, do I have the energy/resources/staff to deal with this tantrum that is about to happen? At the grocery store, on a field trip from school, on the way to a doctor's appointment—at certain moments a parent or teacher will not be able to manage a tantrum or meltdown safely. In such cases it may be best to give the child what he wants or needs at the beginning, avoiding the outburst and avoiding reinforcement of the outburst. If you are working with a child with a significant psychiatric disorder such as autism or a severe anxiety disorder, and the child does not have the cognitive or emotional skills and flexibility to cope with not getting what he wants, it may be best to "give in" to avoid a tantrum, and then work with the child to develop his skills for frustration tolerance and coping with distress.

Once the tantrum starts, the child is likely to become intensely angry. This will likely only last a few minutes, and trying to interact with the child as he is rolling into the anger of an outburst is rarely helpful. Mostly, the best strategy is to back off until the anger peaks and the child shifts into distress. The child feels stressed, helpless, and lost. The transition from anger to distress usually occurs within the 90 seconds of the tantrum, so as a general rule waiting until 2 minutes into the tantrum before trying to intervene can simplify our efforts. In those 2 minutes, ignore the child and pretend to do something–anything–so you do not reinforce the outburst with attention. Keep an ear out for the shift in tone from anger to whimpering or silence.

Listen and Empathize

As anger declines, there will be moments of silence, and moments of fussing and whining, all waxing and waning their way to the end of the outburst. This may take a few minutes or last longer for a child with prolonged tantrums. The goal during this period is to help the child feel understood, and to help him to get back to a calm and regulated state, without reinforcing the negative behaviors of the tantrum with attention or other rewards.

To accomplish this, the moment there is silence, quickly turn to the child, kneel down to his level, look at his face, and read his expression. If he is still sad, try an empathic statement such as "Oh honey, I know you are sad; I get really sad when I don't get to have chocolate whenever I want too; it does seem unfair doesn't it?" while maintaining a sympathetic sad face. For a younger child, you could also speak for the child, in a childlike voice, to identify her emotional state and what made her sad: "Oh, Lara is so sad right now…" By matching the child's experience using both verbal and nonverbal cues, we show that we are attuned to what she is experiencing, which soothes her, reduces her distress (both psychologically and on a hormonal and neurochemical level), and helps her regain balance. We are also helping her to learn to name her emotions and wants for next time. This is more effective than immediately jumping to cheer a child up or distract her with something else, which can be disorienting to the child, does not make her feel understood, and does not teach her to recognize and process her emotions.

If the child appears less sad after an empathic statement, then you can shift to praising and validating the child's return to self-control: "Oh look, you were upset and you did such a good job calming down." A quick comment is sufficient, to reinforce the positive behavior without going overboard and reinforcing the tantrum. Then get back to the task that was interrupted by the tantrum if you can, so that the outburst does not become a useful way to avoid situations or activities that the child dislikes.

Collaborate to Find Solutions

Some children are easily able to express what upset them and triggered a tantrum, but most will need help in determining and articulating the source of their distress. In trying to find the causes of tantrums, remember the ABCs of behavior—the Antecedent, the Behavior, and the Consequence. The **antecedent** is the stage set with its unique environment before the outburst, containing that which is upsetting the child. The **behavior** is the outburst, and the **consequence** is the subsequent situation that supports, or reinforces, the behavior. An important idea here is that the behavior is functional, and that is why it exists and continues. After we figure out the function, we can formulate a hypothesis for behavioral change through modification of factors within our power, including the antecedent and the consequence (Alberto and Troutman 2012).

Even if the child cannot spontaneously volunteer the triggers or antecedents for his tantrum, if you identify and suggest a few possibilities, he will likely be able to identify what it was. Have this discussion once the child has completely calmed down, and be empathic to the fact that he is embarrassed and reluctant to talk about the outburst. If you can help children in these situations feel understood and not judged, you will generally find that even the most disruptive youngsters recognize that tantrums are not the best way to solve problems and are open to help. Once you have identified the antecedent, you can help the child identify an alternative behavior, other than a tantrum, to manage that antecedent. For example, if the child was hungry or he was frustrated because he did not understand the assignment in class, teach him a simple way to express that and get help. (If it is a child with language deficits, a special signal or card that he can hold up for the teacher can be used.) Then you can reinforce this new behavior with a positive consequence—a sticker, token, star, or points toward a larger reward. Even praise or prestige (such as getting to help the teacher) can be a strong reinforcer for positive behavior for many kids. The consequence—for either a positive behavior or a negative one—should be close in time to the behavior, and must be consistently delivered, in order to effectively change a child's behavior.

Learning From the Crisis

Although tantrums are frustrating and disruptive to all involved, they can also be an opportunity to identify when a child's current skills and abilities are not sufficient to cope with a task or situation and where help and teaching is needed. The concept of *scaffolding*–giving support and teaching to reinforce baby steps toward the goal, then removing some of those supports as the child learns the skill–is very useful here. Just as a child learning to read first needs someone to read to him, then read with him, then help him sound out the words, then encourage him to read alone but with the adult right there for help, before he can successfully read on his own, a child learning social skills and self-regulation skills needs the same step-by-step help. The scaffolding process begins with identifying where the skills deficit lies. For example, a child with language deficits who tantrums when he wants to take a break from his schoolwork has several skills deficits. First, he lacks the language skills to ask for a break. Second, he may be having difficulty with the schoolwork and needs academic help (and perhaps help in knowing how to ask for help). Third, he lacks the ability to tolerate frustration if he is not allowed to take a break, and finally, he lacks the ability to delay gratification and keep doing his schoolwork in anticipation of recess later. For this child, the goal is for him to be able to do an entire class period's worth of schoolwork without a break (or a tantrum). However, if we ask this of him now he will not be able to do it. Scaffolding for this child could involve first giving him a few 2-minute break cards that he can raise to request a break; providing additional help with the classwork (perhaps through a 1:1 paraprofessional or tutor); and specifying some work in his speech therapy on asking for help or asking for a break. After a few weeks of this, the next step might be to give a reward if he is able to do 15 minutes of classwork without a break, and do the work without help (or try it without assistance and ask for help if needed), and let him earn greater rewards (favorite activities, privileges, or special treats at home or at school) by going longer and longer without a break and without the 1:1 staff there. By rewarding the use of his new skills and positive behaviors, we help him internalize these skills, so he no longer needs reminders or the immediate support of the 1:1 staff to be able to do what he needs to do. The process is slow and the supports cannot be withdrawn too quickly. When work gets more difficult, or if there is a new stress or difficulty, the tantrums may return, requiring another round of scaffolding.

When to Get Help

There are many resources and successful programs to guide us in helping kids who have frequent tantrums and in preventing disruptive behaviors.

Parenting programs such as Incredible Years, Triple P, and Helping the Noncompliant Child are helpful in decreasing disruptive behavior in children with these problems, often with added benefits such as improvement in parent-child relationship and decrease in parental stress (McGilloway et al. 2012; McMahon and Forehand 2003; Sanders et al. 2000). Common features of successful programs include working with parents on limit setting, time-outs, ignoring, praise, tangible rewards, and problem solving, and helping the parents to understand the child's thinking and behavior (Bernstein et al. 2013). Some programs include other elements such as parent-child relationship building and anger management for the child. Mentoring programs may also benefit children with problems in emotion regulation. In one study, when kindergarten through third-grade students were paired with adult mentors who spent a half hour each week for 14 weeks focusing on modeling, role-playing, and scaffolding to promote use of skills for regulating emotions, teachers reported a 50% decrease in behavior problems (Wyman et al. 2010).

When tantrums are excessive or when programs like those cited above are not working, the child should be referred for evaluation. A behavioral evaluation by the school psychologist is the best first step, as he or she can watch the child in the moment of the tantrum to get the best understanding of the triggers, antecedents, and reinforcers. Even if the child has an outpatient therapist or psychiatrist already, a behavioral evaluation in the school can be immensely valuable. Outpatient clinicians get to see a child for 45 minutes a week at best, and school-based psychologists and social workers can get a much fuller understanding of the child's needs and functioning.

If a child becomes aggressive with herself or others during the tantrum, a referral to an outpatient psychological or psychiatric evaluation and treatment can be useful, and is likely to be more productive than a trip to the ER. Only if the child really cannot be calmed or stabilized is an ER visit the best course of action, and when you do refer a child to the ER, remember that without your observations and descriptions of the behavior, the ER staff will be unable to do much to help the child. By the time the child arrives in the ER, she is usually calm and contrite, and the parents often have no idea what happened and may wonder if the school is pathologizing their child. If the teacher, staff, or counselor who witnessed the tantrum can go to the ER with the child or speak with the ER staff directly, it will allow a more effective evaluation and treatment plan.

References

Alberto PA, Troutman AC: Applied Behavior Analysis for Teachers, 9th Edition. New York, Pearson, 2012

Alsobrook JP II, Pauls DL: A factor analysis of tic symptoms in Gilles de la Tourette's syndrome. Am J Psychiatry 159(2):291–296, 2002

American Psychiatric Association: Diagnostic and Statistical Manual of Mental Disorders, 5th Edition. Arlington, VA, American Psychiatric Association, 2013

Baroni A, Lunsford JR, Luckenbaugh DA, et al: Practitioner review: the assessment of bipolar disorder in children and adolescents. J Child Psychol Psychiatry 50(3):203–215, 2009

Belden AC, Thomson NR, Luby JL: Temper tantrums in healthy versus depressed and disruptive preschoolers: defining tantrum behaviors associated with clinical problems. J Pediatr 152(1):117–122, 2008

Bernstein A, Chorpita BF, Rosenblatt A, et al: Fit of evidence-based treatment components to youths served by wraparound process: a relevance mapping analysis. J Clin Child Adolesc Psychol August 28, 2013 [Epub ahead of print]

Burke JD, Hipwell AE, Loeber R: Dimensions of oppositional defiant disorder as predictors of depression and conduct disorder in preadolescent girls. J Am Acad Child Adolesc Psychiatry 49(5):484–492, 2010

Carlson GA, Potegal M, Margulies D, et al: Rages—what are they and who has them? J Child Adolesc Psychopharmacol 19(3):281–288, 2009

Cheung MY, Shahed J, Jankovic J: Malignant Tourette syndrome. Mov Disord 22(12):1743–1750, 2007

Developmental Disabilities Monitoring Network Surveillance Year 2010 Principal Investigators; Centers for Disease Control and Prevention: Prevalence of autism spectrum disorder among children aged 8 years—autism and developmental disabilities monitoring network, 11 sites, United States, 2010. MMWR Surveill Summ 63(2):1–21, 2014

Goldin RL, Matson JL, Tureck K, et al: A comparison of tantrum behavior profiles in children with ASD, ADHD and comorbid ASD and ADHD. Res Dev Disabil 34(9):2669–2675, 2013

Goodenough FL: Anger in Young Children. Santa Barbara, CA, Greenwood Publishing, 1975

Kim YS, Fombonne E, Koh Y-J, et al: A comparison of DSM-IV pervasive developmental disorder and DSM-5 autism spectrum disorder prevalence in an epidemiologic sample. J Am Acad Child Adolesc Psychiatry 53(5):500–508, 2014

Kochanska G, Coy KC, Murray KT: The development of self-regulation in the first four years of life. Child Dev 72(4):1091–1111, 2001

McGilloway S, Ni Mhaille G, Bywater T, et al: A parenting intervention for childhood behavioral problems: a randomized controlled trial in disadvantaged community-based settings. J Consult Clin Psychol 80(1):116–127, 2012

McMahon RJ, Forehand RL: Helping the Noncompliant Child, 2nd Edition: Family-Based Treatment for Oppositional Behavior. New York, Guilford, 2003

Nock MK, Kazdin AE, Hiripi E, Kessler RC: Lifetime prevalence, correlates, and persistence of oppositional defiant disorder: results from the National Comorbidity Survey Replication. J Child Psychol Psychiatry 48(7):703–713, 2007

Potegal M, Davidson RJ: Temper tantrums in young children, 1: behavioral composition. J Dev Behav Pediatr 24(3):140–147, 2003

Potegal M, Kosorok MR, Davidson RJ: The time course of angry behavior in the temper tantrums of young children. Ann N Y Acad Sci 794:31–45, 1996

Potegal M, Carlson G, Margulies D, et al: Rages or temper tantrums? The behavioral organization, temporal characteristics, and clinical significance of angry-agitated outbursts in child psychiatry inpatients. Child Psychiatry Hum Dev 40(4):621–636, 2009

Qiu P, Yang R, Potegal M: Statistical modeling of the time course of tantrum anger. Ann Appl Stat 3(3):1013–1034, 2009

Roy AK, Klein RG, Angelosante A, et al: Clinical features of young children referred for impairing temper outbursts. J Child Adolesc Psychopharmacol 23(9):588–596, 2013

Sanders MR, Markie-Dadds C, Tully LA, Bor W: The triple P-positive parenting program: a comparison of enhanced, standard, and self-directed behavioral family intervention for parents of children with early onset conduct problems. J Consult Clin Psychol 68(4):624–640, 2000

Sonuga-Barke EJ, Brandeis D, Cortese S, et al: Nonpharmacological interventions for ADHD: systematic review and meta-analyses of randomized controlled trials of dietary and psychological treatments. Am J Psychiatry 170(3):275–289, 2013

Stringaris A, Goodman R: Longitudinal outcome of youth oppositionality: irritable, headstrong, and hurtful behaviors have distinctive predictions. J Am Acad Child Adolesc Psychiatry 48(4):404–412, 2009

Stringaris A, Baroni A, Haimm C, et al: Pediatric bipolar disorder versus severe mood dysregulation: risk for manic episodes on follow-up. J Am Acad Child Adolesc Psychiatry 49(4):397–405, 2010

Tureck K, Matson JL, Cervantes P, Konst MJ: An examination of the relationship between autism spectrum disorder, intellectual functioning, and comorbid symptoms in children. Res Dev Disabil 35(7):1766–1772, 2014

Wakschlag LS, Choi SW, Carter AS, et al: Defining the developmental parameters of temper loss in early childhood: implications for developmental psychopathology. J Child Psychol Psychiatry 53(11):1099–1108, 2012

Wakschlag LS, Briggs-Gowan MJ, Choi SW, et al: Advancing a multidimensional, developmental spectrum approach to preschool disruptive behavior. J Am Acad Child Adolesc Psychiatry 53(1):82–96.e3, 2014

Wickramaratne P, Gameroff MJ, Pilowsky DJ, et al: Children of depressed mothers 1 year after remission of maternal depression: findings from the STAR*D-Child study. Am J Psychiatry 168(6):593–602, 2011

Wyman PA, Cross W, Hendricks Brown C, et al: Intervention to strengthen emotional self-regulation in children with emerging mental health problems: proximal impact on school behavior. J Abnorm Child Psychol 38(5):707–720, 2010

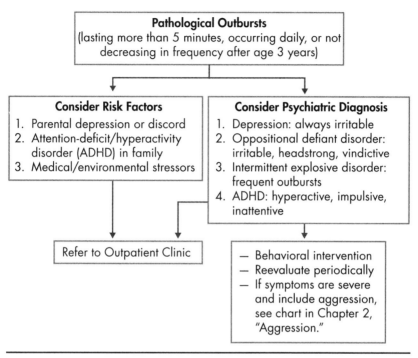

Managing temper tantrums.

CHAPTER 5

The "Odd" Child

Rachel Mandel, M.D.

Every teacher, pediatrician, and therapist can remember a child they have worked with who, while not disruptive or dangerous in any way, was just odd or unusual. Whether it is a child who talks in a constant monotone, or wears the same exact outfit every day, or has bizarre beliefs or interests, it can be difficult to tell where the line is between "quirky" and troubled and know when to refer for help. But the intuition of those who know a child best is incredibly valuable, and often a child who inspires that twinge of concern is falling behind in important age-appropriate developmental, social, and learning milestones. A "quirky" child may have difficulty fitting in in school, may be teased or bullied, may feel isolated and lonely, and may begin to fall behind academically. A child who speaks in a monotone may have undiagnosed autistic spectrum disorder, and one who wears the same clothes every day may be suffering from obsessive-compulsive disorder (OCD) or paranoia, or the child's family may be extremely poor and he may not own other clothing. Such children do not pull for the attention of adults the way an explosive or crying child does, but intervention for them can be just as powerful and put them back on the path to full functioning, even if they will always be "quirky."

Case Presentation

Melissa, a 13-year-old girl, is starting her new school in an eighth-grade Integrated Co-Teaching class. She seems quiet, even indifferent, and bored in class, though never oppositional or disrespectful. She rarely turns in assignments and only shrugs when asked about them. Melissa only raises her hand during class to go to the bathroom, and she does so nearly every period. She does not interact with classmates unless it is part of an assignment, and even then she barely speaks and makes poor eye contact. During free time, she keeps to herself—even at recess, she shows more interest in the trees, flowers, and squirrels than in her peers. One day in class, all of a sudden Melissa becomes despondent and starts crying. She is sent to the counselor's office, where she continues crying for the next half hour, unable to be comforted, only able to intermittently calm down enough to say that she feels "stupid" and "sad" and "I don't understand anything." Given Melissa's level of distress, her mother is called to bring her to the emergency room (ER) for further assessment.

Understanding the Crisis

We tend to spend more time and energy focusing on calming disruptive children to allow for a more peaceful classroom for all students, so quiet children are often overlooked until it is too late. There can be significant distress building up under the outward appearance of calm and shyness. Of course, some children are more introverted by nature, and this is not a problem in and of itself. However, if they are not functioning at the same level as their peers, it is likely having an impact on their self-image and self-esteem and may reflect a significant underlying issue.

In order to understand a sudden outburst like Melissa's, we must first understand the child's usual functioning—why was she behaving so "oddly" in the first place? Is she quiet in all classes or just particular classes? Is she equally introverted at home and during extracurricular activities? Does she seem to be nervous in social situations? Other than the relative lack of speech, does she seem to be like other girls her age, or does she seem to be in her own world? Why doesn't she interact with her peers? Does she want to interact with her peers? How is she doing with her academics? Is something stressful going on at home? Was anything different in her old school?

Getting a sense of a child like Melissa is particularly difficult when the child is new to a school. "Fitting in" can take some time, even for socially adept kids. Important data, like socioemotional history and special needs, can be lost. Even in natural transitions, such as between middle and high schools, communication of crucial information cannot be taken for granted.

When in doubt, the first step is to contact the child's parent for whatever information and documentation he or she can provide. If the concerning behaviors are isolated to school, then the child may be having problems more directly related to school like learning disability or speech pathology. If the parent is noticing similar issues at home, then there could be a more pervasive psychiatric problem present. Talking to the parent can also clarify if this is a change—a reaction to the stress of a new school, or the onset of an anxiety disorder or psychosis—or if the child has always been quiet or different in this way.

A sensitive staff member (be it a teacher, counselor, dean, therapist, or other professional) can learn a lot about an "odd" child by talking or, in the case of younger children, playing with them one-on-one in a safe and supportive environment. Kids like Melissa can seem so challenging and surprising in the course of a normal day, particularly if they have not come to staff attention before, that the initial impulse is often to send them for a psychiatric evaluation emergently. But if kids are able to engage with staff individually and are given the space and time to calm down, they are more likely to open up to a trusted staff person than to a stranger in a frightening ER. Even if the child does not open up completely and share what is wrong, the staff can make observations about the child's behavior, speech, and overall style of interacting that can be very useful for a mental health clinician to know to make a diagnosis. What makes this child seem different from the rest of the class? What makes the child seem similar to the rest of the class?

Melissa was calm by the time she reached the ER. She was a bit tentative at first and embarrassed by what had happened at school. After some neutral, unrelated conversation with staff, she was able to talk about what had been going on at school. In the conversation Melissa mispronounced or misunderstood several words, and she acknowledged being self-conscious about her speech. Melissa's mother told staff that Melissa used to get more help with speech and language in her old school, but those services were not available at her new school, and school was thus much harder for her—at home, Melissa was her normal self. Staff provided information to help secure more services for her in school again. Other than the speech and language difficulties, Melissa presented as a normal 13-year-old girl. Once she felt comfortable with staff, she spoke readily about age-appropriate topics, smiling and making good eye contact. She indeed had friends, but they were mostly old friends in her neighborhood with whom she felt less self-conscious; she talked about wanting to make friends in her new school, but she was nervous about rejection. She also interacted pleasantly and playfully with her mother and younger siblings. Melissa acknowledged feeling overwhelmed in the new, less specialized school setting; she did not understand the work and instruction and did not know where to begin to complete it. She missed the friends and teachers from her old school, and she had not wanted to tell anybody about her struggles because she did not want to disappoint them. She felt like she was trying her hardest every day but it was no use. In today's class review for a major test, she felt hopelessly behind and became preoccupied with the thought of failing and being a disappointment to her family, and this led to her tearful break-down. Melissa was receptive to the staff recommendation of increased speech and language services at school as well as a referral for outpatient therapy for additional support and social skills.

Identifying Kids at Risk

There is such a broad spectrum of "normal" variants in children that it is difficult to know when the "odd" child is of concern. It is important to keep sociocultural factors in mind when thinking about children. Some kids may be ingrained with strict behavioral rules whereby it is considered rude to speak spontaneously or to look an adult in the eye. Some families may believe in ghosts or spirits that they can see or hear. In such contexts, what may present as odd behavior could be entirely normal for this child.

There are also plenty of children who seem awkward but who are happy and healthy and social. Children have a wide array of passions, and unconventional interests are usually not problematic at all. We are all familiar with teenagers dyeing, piercing, and tattooing their bodies and experimenting with different forms of art, music, and literature. There is absolutely nothing inherently wrong with this. There is also nothing necessarily concerning about children who are naturally quiet. In general, the red flags should arise when the child is not functioning well globally, or if there is a sudden change in a child or adolescent's behavior. Even awkward and quiet and eccentric children tend to crave friendships and have the capacity to maintain them. Children with no friends or those with no apparent desire or capacity for social interaction are very worrisome and should be evaluated. Other clues that there could be a significant underlying mental health issue include very narrow interests, not understanding social cues, missing the context in conversation, or not picking up on nonverbal cues in class. Children with these characteristics might be labeled as "problematic kids," who refuse to follow the routine or get into arguments or fights without apparent reason. Closer investigation, however, may reveal that they are reacting to perceived threats to their inflexible thought processes and patterns (Bostic and King 2007).

Differential Diagnosis

There are many reasons for a child to strike us as "odd" that are outside of the range of normal human variations. The following are some common underlying psychiatric disorders in which children present as "odd."

Autism Spectrum Disorder

We used to think of autism as a specific severe disorder whereby children were "stuck in their own world," unable to speak or communicate with other people and doomed to live their lives dependent on caretakers. We now recognize that individuals with autism spectrum disorder can range from those who require round-the-clock assistance for survival to those who flourish in life independently with only more subtle deficits in communication and behavior. As autism spectrum disorder has become more well known and identified, many celebrities, including actors, writers, musicians, and entrepreneurs, have openly discussed their struggles with autism. As the diagnosis becomes less taboo and stigmatizing, there is more awareness of signs and symptoms among parents and those who work with children. Autism is a complicated problem that requires specialized intervention; if autism is suspected, the child's parent should be referred for a comprehensive evaluation for the child as soon as possible, because early intervention is of utmost importance in effective treatment (Dawson et al. 2012).

The key difficulty in autism spectrum disorder lies in social communication. Children with autism spectrum disorder have difficulty with social interaction and can show unusual behaviors such as monotonous or robotic speech, poor eye contact, lack of understanding of social (especially nonverbal) cues, and lack of facial expression. In younger children, we see lack of eye contact and lack of imaginative or make-believe play. Children with autism also often engage in unusual repetitive behaviors, particularly when they are stressed or upset. These behaviors can be intense and troublesome, like head banging and violent rocking or hand flapping, but they are often more subtle, like repeatedly straightening clothing or tapping fingers in a particular sequence. Repetition, ritual, and preoccupation can also be seen in the autistic child's thought process; the child tends to dwell on concrete details and has difficulty being flexible or spontaneous. Transition time might be very difficult for him, and it can be the first or most notable setting where they demonstrate "odd" behaviors. Autism can be harder to diagnose in those with higher IQ, but early recognition is just as important for these children, because it can allow them to function at their full potential (American Psychiatric Association 2013).

It is important to remember that autism spectrum disorder is pervasive, starting in the first years of life (by age 3) and present in all contexts over time. There are no isolated bouts of autism spectrum disorder. If a child is suddenly noted to be quiet and withdrawn in fourth grade, and this is a change from her usual self noted in first through third grade, then an episodic problem like depression is the more likely culprit. A child who seems to be distracted and isolative in math class but engaged and friendly during recess and extracurricular activities is also not likely to be autistic, as we would expect the child to experience social difficulties both in and out of school; perhaps a learning disorder is at play. We should also be careful not to confuse primary language disorders with autism spectrum disorder. This can be confusing because difficulty with age-appropriate use of language can be a primary feature of both diagnoses. However, the overriding social deficits set autism spectrum disorder apart. Children with expressive or receptive language disorder have difficulty communicating verbally (which may lead to self-consciousness and frustration, among other things), but they usually find other ways to compensate, such as pointing, bringing things, or smiling, and they are interested in interacting and playing with others.

As our knowledge base has increased regarding autism spectrum disorder, so have diagnostic assessments and effective treatments. A number of treatments have been developed to improve social interaction skills, language skills, and overall functioning. There are also some medications that can help with aggressive or disturbing behaviors that can be part of autism spectrum disorders. Individuals with autism are eligible for supportive services and accommodations through, in New York, the Committee on Special Education and through state and federal programs that provide therapy and social supports even into adulthood (Matson and Goldin 2014).

Anxiety, Anxiety Disorders, and Obsessive-Compulsive Disorder

Anxiety disorders are among the most common psychiatric disorders seen in children, but they often go unrecognized or misdiagnosed because we can focus more on visible behaviors than what is going on in a child's mind. Kids can also be too embarrassed to talk about anxious thoughts, especially when they know that their worries are not realistic but feel powerless to stop them. Sometimes there is a specific trigger of the anxiety, like the illness of a loved one, their parents' divorce, or an upcoming test. Other times, the anxiety seems to come out of the blue and fails all logic, like with children who suddenly stop talking in school but behave normally at home, or those who must wash their hands many times through the day. An anxious child may bolt from the classroom without warning, while another may be so paralyzed by anxiety that he cannot walk through the school doors. Another may sit silent through the school day, too scared to talk to classmates or raise her hand no matter how much she wants to.

The key to identifying anxiety is to talk to the child one-on-one in a safe environment. More mature or articulate kids can talk about their worries; they can have insight into worries being exaggerated or unrealistic, but the worries persist nonetheless. The term "anxiety" is difficult for children to understand, but most kids understand and can talk about "worry" or "being nervous." Still, some anxiety is not directly related to worry; for example, panic attacks can be hard for kids to recognize and explain. The physical symptoms—having rapid heartbeat or breathing, sweating, feeling hot, feeling nauseous, or suddenly needing to go to the bathroom—are often easiest to identify and discuss. Once kids can identify what they feel physically, an adult can help them counteract these senses by teaching them to do the opposite, like putting cold water on their face if they feel hot or taking deep breaths to calm their fast heart. Making an anxiety-reducing plan can be helpful in and of itself to help the child (and adult) regain a sense of control, because one of the most frightening elements of anxiety is the feeling of being out of control (American Psychiatric Association 2013).

A child's anxiety can be difficult for adults to understand and deal with, because the child seems no longer able to manage things they once did, and the soothing and support that used to help is no longer sufficient to manage the worry. It is important for adults to remember that anxiety is not volitional—it is not simply turned on and off. Kids often try to push worries and unwanted thoughts out of their minds, or seek reassurance from adults, but this effort usually makes the worries come back. The key to treating anxiety is learning gradually to let such thoughts come and go—this is counterintuitive and thus takes time and practice with an experienced therapist, and sometimes medication may also be needed.

Anxiety can manifest in many different ways and can look quite "odd." The presentation of anxiety can range from irritability and volatility to silence and avoidance of any social interaction. Social anxiety is common; it can be isolated and specific to particular situations, such as speaking in front of class or using the public toilet, or it can be more generalized, as a feeling of intense discomfort in any interaction with others. Many children simply freeze in anxiety-provoking situations. For example, they feel utterly unable to respond when called on by a teacher to answer a question, so they remain silent until the teacher moves on to another pupil. Another child with similar anxiety might respond by running out of the room. An older child with anxiety might cut class or use drugs to avoid the anxiety-provoking situation, while another may adopt a defensively aggressive stance so that the teacher is less likely to engage him. A child with separation anxiety who generally appears calm and happy may become utterly uncontrollable when her mother leaves her at school, pushing past staff and trying to run out of the building with no regard for safety. It is important to remember that anxiety disorders are very frustrating for those who suffer them—first because they are intrinsically uncomfortable, and second because many kids (especially as they get older) recognize that their anxious reactions are exaggerated responses to benign stimuli, but they nevertheless feel powerless to stop them (Weisman et al. 2009). A child with OCD may need to repeat certain behaviors over and over, like washing or checking the locks, or writing the same sentence over and over again until it is perfect. This child is also different from a child who is simply neat and orderly, because the obsessions and compulsions take up a lot of time and often upset the child.

Selective mutism and school refusal are two particularly challenging manifestations of anxiety. A selectively mute child has the ability to talk, and does talk in some situations, but is entirely silent in others. A common presentation of selective mutism is a child who will not speak at all in school but speaks regularly at home. Selective mutism can be baffling for peers and teachers but is highly treatable by experienced mental health professionals. School refusal can be more daunting because the child often will absolutely not go to school or will have severe tantrums when brought to school, without any clear-cut reason. A therapist working intensively with the school and the home can gradually get the child to come back to school. These children should not be referred for homeschooling, because this reinforces their worry about school, and the longer a child is out of school, the harder it is to get him or her back (Mulligan and Christner 2012).

Psychosis

School-based clinicians and pediatricians confronted with an odd child often worry about psychosis. Psychosis is very rare in children, but its effects can be devastating, so astute identification and early treatment are important. Chronic psychotic disorders like schizophrenia typically begin in young adulthood, though early signs can sometimes be seen in adolescence. Hallucinations and delusions are the most prominent symptoms of psychosis, but disorganized thinking and behavior—lack of attention to hygiene, social withdrawal, lack of academic participation, and saying or writing things that do not make sense—can also be indicative of psychosis. Whereas autistic, anxious, or inattentive children can have odd thoughts and odd ways of thinking, an adult can usually focus and calm these children and make sense of their thoughts. However, with psychotic children, their thoughts or the organization of their thoughts (e.g., how their thoughts are connected) do not make sense or are not grounded in reality (American Psychiatric Association 2013).

What can be confusing about psychosis is that some symptoms that sound like psychosis can actually be normal. For example, **hallucinations**–"hearing things" or "seeing things" that are not there–are a hallmark of psychosis. However, it is not unusual for children to report "hearing voices" as a way to express their own thoughts. Children can also experience seeing or hearing deceased loved ones in the setting of grief, or describe seeing monsters or ghosts before they fall asleep or when they wake up in the middle of the night. These things are unlikely to be real psychosis. One rule of thumb is that psychosis is disturbing–a child typically does not routinely go about her day and start hearing voices when it is time for a history test or when feeling provoked by a peer. A child who hits a classmate and, when punished, says a voice told him to do it is also unlikely to be truly psychotic. More likely he is trying to avoid punishment. Imaginary friends are also a normal part of development and should not be considered psychosis. Even at older ages, unless the child really does not understand that this imaginary person is not real, imaginary friends are more likely a sign of immaturity or cognitive limitation. Although it can be difficult to draw a clear line, children who are truly hallucinating are usually unable to participate fully in routine classwork and social interactions, as they become preoccupied with what's going on inside of their heads. Distinguishing "normal" from "abnormal" (or feigned) hallucinations is complex, and non–mental health professionals should err on the side of safety and refer these children for psychiatric evaluation. Even if the hallucinations are not due to something like schizophrenia, they may be the result of another psychiatric problem, such as substance abuse or depression, or even a medical illness (Mertin and Hartwig 2004).

Like hallucinations, delusions–fixed strong beliefs in something that is not true or not realistic, which is the other hallmark of psychosis–can be difficult to assess in children and adolescents. There are different types of delusions. Children with **paranoid delusions** can appear fearful, withdrawn, or suspicious and generally are unable to function normally because it is difficult to focus on mundane tasks while genuinely feeling like someone is trying to harm you. It is important to distinguish unreal paranoia from real fears, particularly for children who are being bullied, live in dangerous neighborhoods, or have been through war or assault. **Grandiose delusions** can also be seen in the setting of psychotic or manic illness, wherein children have a hyperinflated sense of self, exaggerated beyond typical childlike imaginary play or adolescent sense of invincibility. Examples of grandiose delusions include, but are not limited to, being a god, demon, or powerful political figure or having special powers, and these children can exhibit bizarre behavior in line with their delusions. Again, it is important to distinguish normal childhood enthusiasm–a child who thinks she will grow up to be president, or a youngster who thinks he is the best basketball player in his neighborhood–from true delusions, like a child who believes she can fly and so attempts to jump off the roof. It is not productive to try to argue with delusional persons about their delusions, because this will only upset them. Rather, adults should provide support in a safe environment while arranging for emergency evaluation. We have several antipsychotic medications and psychotherapeutic techniques to treat psychosis, though it is often part of chronic disorders that will require ongoing support (David et al. 2013).

Attention-Deficit/Hyperactivity Disorder

Attention-deficit/hyperactivity disorder (ADHD) is more than being "hyper." Children with ADHD can seem quite odd because they act on impulses that most children can inhibit. For instance, children with ADHD are often up out of their seat or constantly squirming or fidgeting while sitting. They often speak without raising their hand or before being called on, and their contributions to conversation can be random and off-topic. It can be very difficult for kids with ADHD to make and maintain friends, because other kids can find them annoying. They can be quite clumsy and accident-prone (American Psychiatric Association 2013).

The inattentive form of ADHD is easy to miss, because these children are not as disruptive as those with predominantly hyperactive and impulsive symptoms. Children with primarily inattentive ADHD often seem distracted and quiet, particularly in a large classroom. They have difficulty staying on tasks and completing assignments. They tend to be disorganized, so even if they understand and complete schoolwork, they often leave it at home or lose it somewhere in their locker or backpack. They are forgetful and often lose things (this can be most noticeable in the winter, where inattentive children can misplace many sweaters, gloves, scarves, hats, and even coats). Medications and psychotherapeutic techniques can be very helpful for these kids, as well as for those who are more hyperactive or impulsive. Behavioral strategies and in-school accommodations can also be very helpful. If ADHD is suspected, evaluation at the local mental health clinic should be discussed with parents. ADHD rarely requires emergency evaluation (Spetie and Arnold 2007).

Abuse and Neglect

Children who are being abused or neglected at home may behave strangely at school or with other adults. Children often do not immediately feel comfortable approaching adults about these problems, but odd behaviors can be telling. Children who do not have supportive, caring families at home often mirror these relationships outside of the home. Children who are accustomed to receiving physical violence at home may inflict physical violence upon their peers at school. Alternatively, they may seem detached and fearful, scared of making mistakes or saying the wrong thing. Children with a known history of abuse or neglect may have transitioned through several different foster homes, making stable connections difficult—these children can be reticent in making attachments or can attach too strongly (e.g., hugging adults indiscriminately). Children who seem unkempt and undernourished, who have medical problems that are not attended to, or who steal or dig food out of the trash may be being neglected at home. Abuse and neglect can have very serious and dangerous outcomes for children, and suspected cases should be reported to Child Protective Services immediately—mental health evaluation is not necessary to make a report.

The first priority for abused or neglected children is to ensure their safety. Once they are in a safe environment, psychotherapy can be very helpful in providing an ongoing sense of support and working through past traumas when needed. It is important to recognize that even in cases of severe abuse or neglect, children have a natural desire to be with their biological parents, so removal or separation from the parent is intensely stressful, even if the parent was frankly abusive. Mixed feelings about biological parents and foster parents can last for years, and major life occurrences or anniversaries on either side (e.g., births, deaths, incarcerations, new foster siblings) can stir up ambivalent emotions and changes in behavior (Lau and Weisz 2003).

Substance Abuse

Substance abuse is unfortunately common in high school and middle school students. Different substances are more or less prevalent in different communities, so adults should be familiar with any drug fads in their area. For instance, crystal meth is more prevalent in rural regions, while opiates and cocaine are more common in dense cities. Although alcohol and marijuana have been popular with teenagers for generations, we have seen a steady rise in abuse of prescription medications, such as Oxycontin, Xanax, and Adderall. It is rare for a child to need to carry any type of medication on his or her person in school—medications, particularly controlled substances, are usually kept with the school nurse—so a child observed with pills on him should be investigated. Newer synthetic drugs have also become popular with kids because they are often initially sold legally and may be undetected by drug screens (Kelly et al. 2013). The effects of these substances, such as K2 and "bath salts," can be unpredictable and dangerous. The typical presentations of intoxication and withdrawal from common substances of abuse are discussed in Chapter 9, "Substance Use."

Learning, Language, and Intellectual Disabilities

Undiagnosed learning, language, and intellectual disabilities can be devastating for children. They can feel out of place in a classroom that is not suited to their needs, and they fall farther behind each year that their needs are not addressed. These disabilities can often be diagnosed and remediated at a young age, but lack of knowledge and resources among parents and schools can often delay this process for years. Some children act out aggressively in response, but many simply stay silent and pass along year after year, though it is very difficult for them to make it all the way through high school without accommodations. Even as early as kindergarten, these children can be aware of their limitations and feel different from their peers—they are often reticent in class and afraid to ask questions.

Teachers are in the unique position of gauging a child's academic performance and progress with their class and with community standards or expectations. A child may have a disability in a specific academic area or in several. A teacher who suspects that a student has a disability should discuss this with the student's parents. These difficulties are often present from early childhood, though they can become more prominent with age as academics become more complicated (e.g., a child with a reading disorder may have much more difficulty once she reaches middle school and all subjects require significant reading). The teacher can recommend that the parent request a psychoeducational evaluation from the school to determine if the child has any disabilities and, if so, what accommodations can be provided. Repeating a grade for academic failures should be considered a red flag for learning, language, or intellectual disability, and a psychoeducational evaluation should be considered. It is important to note that these children often do not seem "dumb"—they can be socially adept, articulate, and clever in nonacademic settings. Many have struggled with their deficits for most of their lives and have adapted to get through the school day and stay under the radar. Still, the academic work is what tells the true story. Avoidant behaviors, like needing to go to the nurse or the bathroom during certain classes, should also be noted (Willcutt and Pennington 2000).

Risk Assessment

It can be difficult to decide what to do with an "odd" child. As always, if the child is posing any immediate danger to himself or others, 911 should be called. Psychotic symptoms should also be evaluated emergently even if there is not an obviously dangerous situation present, because a child who is not grounded in reality can unwittingly put himself in danger, and because psychosis is toxic to the brain and should be treated as soon as possible. Ongoing behaviors that are simply odd and not dangerous are a different story. A good rule of thumb is that sudden changes require more immediate attention because we should figure out what acutely caused the change and treat it; this could be the case in substance abuse. More stable and consistent "oddness" should be addressed when it causes the child distress or social problems as in autism spectrum disorder, anxiety disorders, OCD, or ADHD; parents should be consulted about arranging an outpatient mental health assessment. "Oddness" that seems related to academic struggles should be discussed with parents to make a referral for psychoeducational testing as soon as possible. Most adults who work with children are mandated reporters of abuse and neglect, and any suspicions of abuse or neglect should be reported to Child Protective Services immediately. Further outpatient psychotherapy services can be arranged once the child's safety is ensured.

Onsite Stabilization

No matter what the suspected diagnosis is, it is most important that all children feel safe and supported. It can be particularly difficult for "odd" children to make friends and feel welcomed in schools, so it is important that staff be available and reach out to these children, even outside of a crisis moment. For children with anxiety, autism, or social difficulties, when stressed or upset they can often be comforted by some free time with a trusted teacher or counselor, or a calming activity, with the ultimate goal of rejoining their peers or the classroom. If emergency medical services (EMS) is required, as in the case of a psychotic or intoxicated child, the child should be kept in a safe area, monitored by a trusted adult, without other children present. Offer words of support–do not attempt to disprove disordered thoughts, delusions, or hallucinations, as this may be perceived as more threatening. Talk directly and simply, so that the child has a good opportunity to cooperate–this is not the time for a series of whys. While waiting for EMS to arrive, it is often most effective to address the child's immediate concrete needs, perhaps a snack or drink or a phone call home. We do not want to reward behavioral outbursts (we have all seen angry teenagers demanding cell phones and video games), but if there is a particular activity or interest that is known to be soothing to the child, it can be effectively utilized. This is especially true for children with autism spectrum disorder who have specific narrow interests.

Catch the Warning Signs

As discussed throughout this chapter, there are a number of possible contributors to the "oddness" of a child, ranging from mild autism to severe psychosis. Trying to understand the child, what is going on with her, what her difficulties are, and what things tend to upset her in advance can help you to prevent a crisis. For example, children with milder autistic or anxiety symptoms may function quite well most of the time but struggle with change in routine or structure. When such changes can be anticipated and approached gradually with the child, a crisis is often avoided. If changes come by surprise and a crisis does ensue, think about what things the child likes and what she may find calming and soothing. Children approaching crisis often feel out of control—helping them to regain their sense of self-control can avert a crisis before it begins.

Listen and Empathize

It can seem impossible to know what is going on with an "odd" child. Sometimes the child can tell you exactly what is bothering her, and sometimes she can be utterly perplexed as to why you are bothering her at all. The most important thing for an adult to do is to create a safe and supportive environment for the child to take advantage of as needed. If the child is able and willing to talk to you, try to see the situation from her perspective. It does not matter if her thinking makes sense to you; you are just trying to understand from her vantage point. Children are not used to adults truly listening, so sometimes just that is enough to help a child calm down.

Collaborate to Find Solutions

It can be difficult for any child to express verbally what she needs, and this is particularly true for children with autism or other social skills problems, learning disabilities, anxiety disorders, or other difficulties. A child with social deficits will likely have as much trouble expressing herself to an adult as to a peer. However, an adult can provide more time and patience, which will hopefully allow for more openness down the line. After listening to and beginning to understand the child's perspective, adults can offer potential solutions both to avoid meltdowns and to increase the child's ability to function normally in the future. This may mean a counseling session where a child can get her anxieties off of her chest and practice relaxation strategies. More often, it is an empty classroom where a child can eat lunch and read a book without navigating baffling cafeteria politics. The ultimate goal is for the child to have enough comfort and social skills to reintegrate with her same-age peers, but this is a long process. A child who has difficulty communicating verbally may be more able to do so in a non-judgmental one-on-one setting, but such a setting could also serve as a break for a struggling child to play cards or a board game–to interact more concretely and thus feel empathy without the need for words.

Learning From the Crisis

It is imperative to review crisis events after the child is fully calm in order to figure out how to help most effectively in the long term. If the child was sent for emergency, outpatient, or inpatient psychiatric assessment, ask the parent for any discharge summary, diagnosis, or recommendations provided by the mental health clinician. The family's right to privacy must be respected, but any information that can be shared with staff could be useful in developing a more supportive environment for the child. The child should also be addressed individually to reflect on the crisis, both to provide staff with a subjective account of events and to hear staff's observations. Whenever possible, triggers to the crisis should be identified, and alternative responses should be explored. If psychoeducational testing, Individualized Education Programs (IEPs), 504 accommodations, or behavioral plans are recommended, then these should be discussed with the child at an age-appropriate level so that such changes do not come as a surprise. In fact, such changes can often be a relief to a child who is struggling.

When to Get Help

All of the mental health problems described in this chapter have effective treatments. Unfortunately, many of our medications and therapies take months to really work, and many of our clinics have long wait lists. Similarly, the process for psychoeducational referral, testing, and IEP development and, finally, implementation can take the better part of a school year. Thus, quick identification of problems and discussion with parents for mental health referral are crucial for recovery. Again, there is no clear barometer for what level of "oddness" necessitates psychiatric evaluation–the best measure is the child's overall level of functioning (social, academic, and emotional) as compared with his or her same-age peers. Children are certainly allowed to be quiet and awkward, but children who are isolated and struggling to keep up are often in significant distress.

If you do refer a child for psychiatric evaluation, either in a clinic or to an ER, remember that your insights and observations can be hugely helpful to the clinician seeing the child. Send a referral letter expressing your concerns and give your phone number so the clinician can call you directly. If there is a child you are really worried about and the first doctor says, "It's nothing," it may be that the doctor is not seeing everything that you see (particularly if he or she has only had a short time with the child). Share your concerns, or seek a second opinion.

References

American Psychiatric Association: Diagnostic and Statistical Manual of Mental Disorders, 5th Edition. Arlington, VA, American Psychiatric Association, 2013

Bostic J, King R: Clinical assessment of children and adolescents: content and structure (Chapter 4.2.2), in Lewis's Child and Adolescent Psychiatry: A Comprehensive Textbook, 4th Edition. Edited by Martin A, Volkmar FR. Philadelphia, PA, Lippincott Williams & Wilkins, 2007, pp 323–344

David CN, Gogtay N, Rapoport JL: Early schizophrenia and psychotic illnesses, in Clinical Manual of Child and Adolescent Psychopharmacology, 2nd Edition. Edited by McVoy M, Findling RL. Washington, DC, American Psychiatric Publishing, 2013, pp 347–395

Dawson G, Jones E, Merkle K: Early behavioral intervention is associated with normalized brain activity in young children with autism. J Am Acad Child Adolesc Psychiatry 51(11):1150–1159, 2012

Kelly B, Wells B, Pawson M, et al: Novel psychoactive drug use among younger adults involved in US nightlife scenes. Drug Alcohol Rev 32(6):588–593, 2013

Lau A, Weisz J: Reported maltreatment among clinic-referred children: implications for presenting problems, treatment attrition, and long-term outcomes. J Am Acad Child Adolesc Psychiatry 42(11):1327–1334, 2003

Matson J, Goldin R: Early intensive behavioral interventions: selecting behaviors for treatment and assessing treatment effectiveness. Research in Autism Spectrum Disorders 8(2):138–142, 2014

Mertin P, Hartwig S: Auditory hallucinations in nonpsychotic children: diagnostic considerations. Child and Adolescent Mental Health 9(1):9–14, 2004

Mulligan CA, Christner RW: Selective mutism: cognitive-behavioral assessment and intervention, in Cognitive-Behavioral Interventions in Educational Settings: A Handbook for Practice. Edited by Mennuti RB, Christner RW, Freeman A, Beck JS. New York, Routledge/Taylor & Francis Group, 2012, pp 187–214

Spetie L, Arnold E: Attention-deficit/hyperactivity disorder (Chapter 5.2.1), in Lewis's Child and Adolescent Psychiatry: A Comprehensive Textbook, 4th Edition. Edited by Martin A, Volkmar FR. Philadelphia, PA, Lippincott Williams & Wilkins, 2007, pp 430–454

Weisman A, Antinoro D, Chu B: Cognitive-behavioral therapy for anxious youth in school settings: advances and challenges, in Cognitive-Behavioral Interventions for Emotional and Behavioral Disorders. Edited by Mayer MJ, Van Acker R, Lochman JE, Gresham FM. New York, Guilford, 2009, pp 173–203

Willcutt E, Pennington B: Psychiatric comorbidity in children and adolescents with reading disability. J Am Acad Child Adolesc Psychiatry 41(8):1039–1048, 2000

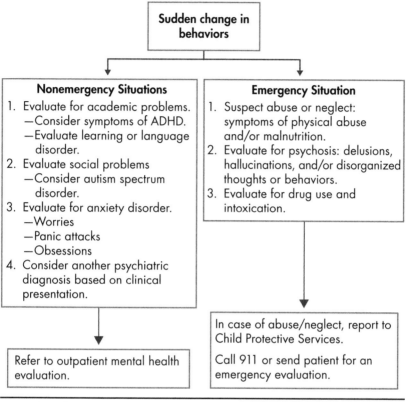

Managing the "odd" child.

CHAPTER 6

Child Abuse and Trauma

Ruth Gerson, M.D.

Each year, more than six million children experience physical or sexual abuse or neglect, and close to two thousand children die from this abuse (U.S. Department of Health and Human Services 2010). One in four children will experience a major trauma before they turn 16—either child abuse or physical or sexual assault; domestic violence; witnessed violence in his or her community; severe bullying; a terrifying accident or sudden loss; a natural disaster; or an act of terrorism (Costello et al. 2002).

The effects of such traumatic experiences on a child can be profound. Many children who have experienced trauma will go on to suffer from depression, anxiety, sleep problems, and problems with attention and behavior. They can be at increased risk for risk-taking behaviors, drug and alcohol use, teen pregnancy, dropping out of school, and criminal behaviors (Gerson and Rappaport 2013). With the right support and treatment, however, traumatized children and adolescents can find a way to understand what has happened to them and put it behind them, to lead healthy and happy lives. Teachers, school mental health providers, and pediatricians can play a critical role in helping to ensure safety for these children and get them the help they need.

Case Presentation

Destiny, a tenth grader in regular education, always used to love school. But this year, she has started fighting with her mother ever morning, refusing to go. When Destiny does go to school, she has dark circles under her eyes, and a few times she has smelled of marijuana. She is sullen and irritable and pays little attention in class. Once one of the stars of the softball team, Destiny dropped the sport a few weeks into the school year, and in the evenings and weekends she just stays in her room, shrugging her mother off in irritation whenever her mom asks if she is okay. Destiny's former softball coach, with whom Destiny had been close before she quit the team, pulls her aside one day after school. Destiny is initially terse, keeping her eyes downcast, but eventually she admits that she has been having trouble sleeping and has been skipping school because leaving her home makes her feel "on edge." In a quiet voice, she tells the coach that a few months ago, on her way home from school, some older boys from the rival high school cornered her, pulled her into an alley, and forced her to perform fellatio on one of them. She has not told her mother because she does not want to upset her. Her mother has been under enough stress ever since her stepfather, newly unemployed, started drinking again. Although her stepfather is normally a nice guy, when he drinks he is unpredictable and explosive, and Destiny worries about her mom. Suddenly tearful, she begs the coach not to tell anyone.

Understanding the Crisis

Abused kids like Destiny always pull at our heartstrings. But before Destiny told her coach what had happened to her, she was just another sullen, irritable kid, smoking marijuana and refusing to go to school. Sometimes kids who have been abused or traumatized will tell us, but more often they are ashamed and keep it secret, while the trauma eats away at them inside and manifests outside as negative behaviors or changes in mood. There are red flags in Destiny's story that make her different from other "bad" kids, and to help a kid like Destiny, it is important that we see through her behaviors, pick up on the warning signs, and try to learn what is really going on.

Youths who have experienced trauma can demonstrate a number of behavioral problems that bring them to the attention of therapists or school administrators or that bring parents to the pediatrician's office asking for help. These behaviors are related to the two natural and automatic reactions that the human body has to a life-threatening event. The **fight-or-flight response** (hereafter referred to as fight-or-flight response) is well known: the body prepares to fight back or to run, with adrenaline pumping, blood flowing to the muscles, and sharpening of the senses and attention. The second common reaction to trauma, the **freeze response,** is less familiar and is rooted in a different neurochemical pathway. A child whose life is in danger, like a deer in the headlights of an oncoming car, will often freeze, both physically and mentally. She is immobile, her ability to speak or process language and to form conscious memories is inhibited, and she feels numb, dissociated (unreal or disconnected), or separated from her body. In these two reactions–fight-or-flight or freeze–we can see the roots of the problem behaviors that are so common in traumatized children and adolescents. With Destiny, for example, her social withdrawal, inattention in class, reluctance to leave her home, and even her marijuana use can be thought of as avoidance behaviors that are part of the freeze response. Destiny says that during her assault, she felt unable to move or fight back and felt separated from her body, like she was watching from above. Since then she has felt numb and distracted, like she is still far away from what is happening in her life, but if she thinks about what happened or experiences any reminder (or **trigger**) of her trauma, she immediately feels overwhelmed with panic and fear.

Another child might become hyperactive and aggressive after a traumatic experience. For example, Destiny's younger stepbrother Eric, who was previously a sweet kid, has been acting up in school ever since he witnessed his intoxicated father beat up Destiny's mom. Watching this assault, Eric experienced the urge to fight–to try to stop the assault–or to run out of the house. Since that incident, he cannot stay in class, and the slightest word from another kid or teacher leads to him cursing, screaming, and throwing things. Just as Destiny's avoidance is an extension of her freeze response, Eric's dysregulation is an extension of his fight-or-flight response.

Girls, young children, and individuals who are experiencing ongoing trauma are more likely to experience the freeze response; whereas boys, older children, and individuals who have witnessed or experienced violence are more likely to manifest the fight-or-flight response (American Academy of Pediatrics 2013). Some children and adolescents, particularly those who have experienced multiple traumas, can alternate between the two responses, appearing numb, shut down, or dissociated (the freeze response) much of the time but becoming extremely agitated, anxious, or aggressive (the fight-or-flight response) when faced with a trauma trigger. These trauma reactions are often confused with other psychiatric illnesses, particularly if adults are not aware that a child has been through a traumatic event. For example, the fight-or-flight response can look like attention-deficit/hyperactivity disorder (ADHD), oppositionality, or anger problems. The freeze response can look like depression or inattentive-type

ADHD, and youths who alternate between freezing and fight-or-flight are often labeled as bipolar or even psychotic. When these types of symptoms come up suddenly in a child or teen, adults should ask carefully about trauma to make sure that the fight-or-flight or freeze response is not at play.

It is also crucial to consider how **context** can lead to problem behaviors in traumatized kids. For example, a child who is being neglected at home may be chronically hungry, and irritable and inattentive as a result; when another kid teases him for being smelly and dirty, this child might become agitated and aggressive. An adolescent girl who has been sexually abused by her stepfather may stay up all night in fear and then in school appear irritable and sleep through class. Children who have been traumatized can also be triggered by things in their environment—meaning that things in the environment remind them of the traumatic experience and bring back the fight-or-flight or freeze response. For example, an elementary school child who experienced a home invasion when home alone with his babysitter may become intensely frightened during a safety drill at school, if the need to hide and stay quiet makes him feel like he is in danger again. A young girl who was physically abused by her stepfather may be fearful of men she does not know, and so she may freeze or run when approached by male staff at her afterschool program. If there is a sudden shift in a child's manner or behavior, if a child's reaction seems out of proportion to the issue at hand, or if a child becomes upset repeatedly when faced with a certain person or situation, he or she may be responding to a trauma trigger. Stepping back and observing the child's behavior and the context for that behavior objectively and dispassionately can help to identify what the trigger might be.

Identifying Traumatized Kids and Those at Risk for Maltreatment

Although everyone who works with children and adolescents knows to look out for child maltreatment (physical, sexual, or emotional abuse or neglect), it can be hard to know which kids to watch. Maltreatment is not the only type of traumatic experience that a child or adolescent can experience. Many of our youths grow up in neighborhoods plagued by community violence, witness domestic violence in their homes, experience bullying in schools, or experience a personal or community tragedy like a fatal car accident, natural disaster, or mass shooting. Not all children will develop psychiatric symptoms after these traumatic events, but every child needs support, caring, and close monitoring after such an experience.

A number of factors put children at risk for maltreatment (Table 6–1), including environmental or family factors and even characteristics of the child himself or herself (Flaherty et al. 2010). Children growing up in families that are poor and without a strong extended family or social network are at increased risk for maltreatment, as are those whose parents are unemployed or struggling with domestic violence or substance abuse, or are teen parents. Parents who have been abused themselves as children, or who struggle with depression or other mental illness, are also more likely to harm their own children or to fail to supervise their children, thus leaving the children susceptible to others who might harm them. Finally, factors in the child–such as physical disabilities or chronic illness, developmental disabilities, or emotional or behavioral problems–can also put a child at greater risk for maltreatment.

TABLE 6–1. Risk factors and red flags for abuse, maltreatment, and trauma

Risk factors for abuse and maltreatment	Physical or intellectual disability
	Emotional or behavioral problems
	Poverty and other severe family stressors
	Foster care placement
	Living in a dangerous or violent community
Red flags that abuse or trauma has occurred	Physical signs
	Unexplained bruises, injuries, or burns
	Poor hygiene, dirty clothes
	Unmet medical needs
	Poor nutrition/emaciation
	Behavioral signs
	Sudden change in behavior
	Onset of symptoms such as hyperactivity, aggression, withdrawal, self-injurious behavior, truancy

Children in foster care and special-needs children are at particularly high risk for abuse. Children in foster care have been removed from their parents because of abuse or neglect, or they have experienced the death of a parent and all of the stress and disruption that comes along with such a traumatic loss. Often children manifest the stress of these early experiences, and the stress of suddenly being placed in a new family, through oppositional behaviors, tantrums, bedwetting, and other regressive behaviors that may be stressful for the foster family and increase the risk that the children are abused again. Children with intellectual and developmental disabilities are at increased risk as well, in part because raising a child with special needs can put a serious strain, both emotional and financial, on parents and increase the risk of abuse or neglect, and also because children with special needs may be targeted by abusers because they are less likely or able to speak up or stop the abuse.

If you have identified a child at risk for maltreatment, there are a number of warning signs that suggest that abuse or neglect may be occurring. Most professionals working with children know to look for physical signs: unexplained bruises, injuries, or burns suggest abuse, while poor hygiene and dirty clothes, an emaciated appearance, and unmet medical needs suggest possible neglect. But there are behavioral signs of abuse and neglect as well. If a child who had previously been well behaved in school returns from the summer vacation suddenly hyperactive, aggressive, angry, or withdrawn, suddenly begins to engage in promiscuous or hypersexual behaviors, shirks physical contact with others, or starts cutting herself, this should raise concern that the child may have been abused. Children who seem not to want to go home from school, or those who are chronically truant, delinquent, or using alcohol or drugs, may be coming from homes where they feel unsafe or where they are not getting appropriate caretaking and supervision. These red flags are not always signs of abuse–there are, of course, children who are truant, use alcohol, or become withdrawn or angry for other reasons. But when a child or teen manifests these behaviors, it is best not to just take it at face value but rather to look deeper to see if there is something else that is having an impact on the child's behavior.

Differential Diagnosis

After a traumatic experience, many children and adolescents will be more anxious, emotional, and clingy; have trouble sleeping; or have nightmares. For many these states will pass, but some children will develop persistent psychiatric symptoms.

Posttraumatic Stress Disorder

After a traumatic event, some children and adolescents will develop posttraumatic stress disorder (PTSD). PTSD was, prior to DSM-5 (American Psychiatric Association 2013), classified as a type of anxiety disorder, but it also affects a child's behavior, memory, and mood. It is now grouped among the trauma- and stressor-related disorders. The symptoms of PTSD fall into four clusters. **Intrusion symptoms,** the first cluster, includes nightmares, flashbacks, intrusive thoughts of the trauma, feeling like the trauma is happening again, or feeling frightened or distressed when reminded of the trauma. Adolescents can usually describe these symptoms fairly clearly, but young children may have a harder time describing flash-backs or intrusive thoughts. Sometimes a young child will instead act out the traumatic experience in her play over and over, or may have night-mares but be unable to say if they are related to the trauma.

The second cluster of PTSD symptoms is characterized by **avoidance.** Children and teens who have experienced trauma or abuse do not want to talk about what happened, or even think about what happened. This is not denial or their being difficult, but rather a reflection of how acutely painful and stressful—emotionally and even physically—these memories are. Ado-lescents can often acknowledge that they are avoiding thinking or talking about it, but children often lack that self-awareness and will simply shut down, say "I don't know," or even deny that anything happened when asked about the trauma.

The third cluster of PTSD symptoms involves **changes in mood and thinking.** Many children with PTSD can appear depressed, with low mood and ruminative thoughts in which they blame themselves for the traumatic event; others are angry or afraid all the time.

The fourth cluster of symptoms, related to the third cluster, involves **marked changes in arousal and reactivity.** Children are often persis-tently irritable, have poor concentration, and sleep poorly (because of night-mares, fear of falling asleep, or restless sleep), and are chronically "keyed up"—hypervigilant, anxious, and easily startled. Finally, some children, particularly younger children and girls who have experienced repeated trauma, will manifest a dissociative response, with detachment, numbing, and even feelings of "not being real" or "being outside of my body" that can sound almost psychotic but are instead a fairly typical reaction to extreme stress.

One difficulty with making a diagnosis of PTSD is that it can look very different in young children (or older children with intellectual or develop-mental disabilities) from the way it looks in adults or even in adolescents. For young children with PTSD, it is more likely that they will show the emotional and behavioral symptoms—being very anxious or irritable, hav-ing difficulty sleeping, having nightmares, experiencing concentration problems—of PTSD or start to show developmental regression, such as having more tantrums or starting to wet the bed again.

Another difficulty with PTSD is that it can look like other psychiatric disorders, particularly if no one is aware that a trauma has occurred. A young child who has poor concentration and jumps out of his seat every time the male assistant principal comes by might have ADHD—or he could be experiencing abuse from his stepfather at home, having flashbacks, and experiencing male staff as frightening. An adolescent like Destiny in our case example might be diagnosed with bipolar disorder, or her symptoms might be attributed to drug use and conduct problems, when in fact they may be accounted for by PTSD. In order to make the correct diagnosis, mental health professionals should collect as much information as possible about the pattern of the child's behavior and any triggers or precipitants.

Depression and Bipolar Disorder

Depression is one of the most common psychiatric consequences of trauma. In young children, this can manifest as frequent crying, sleep problems such as insomnia or hypersomnia (sleeping too much), lack of enjoyment of favorite activities that may look like fatigue or apathy, or even irritability. Adolescents may be more able to articulate feeling sad, or may describe feeling disconnected from others, numb, or hopeless. Youths who are depressed after a traumatic event often feel guilty and blame themselves for what happened. It is important to monitor carefully for depression after a traumatic event, because depressed youths are at very high risk for suicide and self-injurious behaviors if they do not get proper treatment. Particularly if a young person has newly disclosed abuse or maltreatment, she may feel deeply ashamed and turn to self-harm or suicide. Depression in traumatized youths is less likely to respond to simple talk therapy and may require special trauma-focused therapy and often medication.

Children with PTSD and depression are often misdiagnosed as having bipolar disorder. An adolescent with depression and PTSD is likely to have depressed and irritable mood and sleep problems (both insomnia and nightmares) and, when faced with trauma reminders, may have a sudden change in mood or behavior (e.g., becoming angry or aggressive, having a flashback) that the adolescent and parent may describe as "mood swings." It is important to remember, though, that "mood swings" are not bipolar. When an adolescent (or very, very rarely a child) has bipolar disorder, he has clear episodes of mania (irritability or euphoric mood, decreased sleep, increased spending or hypersexual behaviors, high energy, racing thoughts, and even grandiose delusions) lasting at least a few days. "Mood swings" occurring over the course of the day are very common in adolescents, particularly in traumatized adolescents, and are not a feature of bipolar disorder. That said, children with bipolar disorder can experience trauma and can develop PTSD as a result. A careful history, determining what symptoms started before or after the trauma, can help you parse this out.

Anxiety and Anxiety Disorders

Children who have experienced trauma, including those who develop PTSD, are at risk for anxiety disorders. Separation anxiety is common in young children after a traumatic event, particularly if the child perceived the parent to be in danger in any way (such as in cases of domestic violence, or after an accident). Separation anxiety after trauma can look like school refusal, because the child may fear that the parent could be harmed while she is at school. Young children may also experience night terrors– fits of screaming and panic at night in which they may appear to be awake but are not aware of their surroundings. Panic attacks are more common in older children and adolescents; they may also experience somatic symptoms of anxiety, such as frequent headaches or stomachaches with no physical cause.

Substance Use

Like Destiny in the case example, youths who have experienced trauma are at greatly increased risk for starting to use drugs and alcohol and for using drugs and alcohol at an earlier age and in more risky ways. Adolescents who have experienced physical or sexual abuse are 12 times more likely than nonabused adolescents to start using marijuana or alcohol regularly before the age of 10 (Bensley et al. 1999). Teens with PTSD from other causes are at high risk as well; more than half of teens with PTSD go on to develop problematic drug or alcohol use. They may start using drugs or alcohol to get relief from PTSD symptoms, depression, or anxiety, or they may first take a drink or pill socially and then keep using because the drug is the only thing that makes them feel "normal" again. Adolescents are used to adults condemning their substance use, so if you try to understand why they are using, and what benefit the drug or alcohol has for them, they are much more likely to open up to you about their symptoms and, in turn, be open to finding alternative ways to manage their pain.

Psychosis

It is not uncommon for children who are in foster care, children who have been abused or severely neglected, or children who have recently experienced a traumatic event to be brought to a psychiatrist for "hearing voices." While a very small number of adolescents can develop psychosis after a severe trauma, the majority of children brought in for evaluation do not have psychosis. PTSD flashbacks, intrusive memories, and other reexperiencing symptoms often masquerade as "voices" or as visual hallucinations, particularly in young children with cognitive or language disabilities who have difficulty describing their experience clearly. In children who seem to be hearing or seeing things that are not there, or who seem to be acting in bizarre ways, it is statistically much more likely that they have experienced a traumatic event than that they have a psychotic illness such as schizophrenia.

Attention-Deficit/Hyperactivity Disorder

As noted earlier, children who have experienced abuse or other trauma can look like they have ADHD when in fact they have PTSD. For example, if an adolescent girl has been sexually assaulted by a boy in her school, she may appear inattentive in class due to hypervigilance, always looking at the door to see if the boy is around, or due to reexperiencing and flashback symptoms. But it is important not to automatically attribute everything to the trauma. Children with ADHD are at increased risk for physical abuse (their impulsivity and hyperactivity can make them difficult for parents to manage, so a parent may be more likely to use excessive physical discipline) and for accidents and other traumatic experiences (their impulsivity and poor judgment can get them into dangerous situations). When you are assessing for ADHD symptoms, it is important to ask if the inattention and hyperactivity only started since the trauma, in which case it may be PTSD, or if it started long before the trauma, in which case it is likely "true" ADHD.

Identifying Immediate Triggers

A child or adolescent who has been through a traumatic experience, particularly if he is struggling with one of the disorders just described, will be vulnerable to being triggered by things in his environment. It may not be immediately obvious to adults working with the child when a reminder of the trauma has triggered flashbacks, intrusive memories of the trauma, or automatic behaviors such as fighting, freezing, or fleeing. Unfortunately, it is difficult for kids to tell us when this is happening. Trauma reminders trigger sudden changes in blood flow in the brain so that the language centers of the brain do not get any blood flow or nutrients–so an acutely traumatized child cannot "use his words" to describe what he is experiencing. Even after the fact, it will be difficult for the child to articulate what has upset him; a self-aware adolescent might be able to do so, but the effects of trauma on cognition and memory mean most teens will struggle to recall and describe their triggers.

Trauma triggers may not be obvious. For example, holidays, birthdays, and other happy occasions are often triggers for children who have been removed from their parents because of abuse or neglect. Moving to a new foster home or being returned to live with family, even if it is what the child has wanted, can trigger bad memories and changes in behavior. Traumatized children can also overreact to and misinterpret things in their environment. Adults shouting with excitement or even just talking loudly might sound as if they are yelling and trigger flashbacks of domestic violence at home. If another child in a classroom or pediatrics clinic is having a meltdown and has to be physically held for safety, a child who has been physically or sexually abused is likely to become agitated and even aggressive, as he cannot distinguish in that moment the safe physical contact from the abuse in his memory. Adults working with traumatized children must pay very close attention to what is going on before a child becomes symptomatic, because by identifying patterns we can learn what a child's triggers are and then work to remove them and help the child to learn to cope with them.

Risk Assessment

If you suspect a child has been through a traumatic experience, the most important and first step is ensuring that she is safe, in this moment, at home, at school, and in her community. A child who comes to school with unexplained bruises, burns, or injuries (or with physical symptoms concerning for a sexually transmitted disease); who appears fearful of a parent or babysitter; who is suddenly terrified of physical contact—it may not be safe for this child to leave your office. And it is crucial to ask outright about abuse, as many children will not volunteer information about abuse because they are ashamed, frightened, or worried about getting in trouble. If a child tells you that abuse or violence has happened at home, you must make sure it is not still going on and take action to prevent it from happening again, which may mean calling Child Protective Services (CPS). If the danger is not in the home—for example, if a teenage boy is being threatened by gang members in his building, or if a girl who has been sexually assaulted is being followed by her abuser—it is imperative that you tell the parents and, if necessary, notify the police. Adolescents will often beg you not to tell their parents because they feel like it is their fault, that their parents will be mad, or that somehow their parents could be in danger (like a girl who fears her father will try to kill her rapist). These adolescents will be upset but will understand if you explain to them why you have to tell their parents and what is going to happen. It can also help to give them some sense of control—do we tell your parents together, or would you prefer that I tell them alone? Do you want to say the words and I will listen, or would it help if I say it for you? By staying calm and in control, even if the child gets upset or angry at you, you are showing that you can and will keep him safe. Sometimes the trauma is something that the child and family have gone through together—a home invasion, an abusive stepfather, a terrifying fire leading to sudden homelessness, a threat of deportation for an undocumented family—and in those cases you can work together with the parents to understand the child's reaction and ensure everyone is safe.

After evaluating whether the environment is safe, think about whether it is healthy—an environment that is full of trauma reminders and triggers is going to be almost as disruptive to a child's well-being as one where trauma is ongoing. Parents and other caretakers may not realize how trauma reminders can impact a child. For example, if a young boy has been sexually abused, the parent may push to press charges, assuming that the child will feel better working to get the perpetrator locked away. But for many young victims of abuse, being interviewed by police, testifying in front of judges, and feeling fearful about confronting their perpetrator in the courtroom can feel like a second trauma, particularly if there are not the right therapeutic supports in place to help get them through it. If a child has been abused by her parent and is now in foster care, visits from the foster care agency or supervised sessions with the parent can trigger posttraumatic stress symptoms or changes in behavior or mood. Even simple things like bedtime can remind the child of the abusive parent—because either that was a time that the child was often hurt or that was one of the few nice moments the child would have with the parent. Adults sometimes expect that a child will be "fine' as soon as she is removed from the immediate danger and do not realize how the effects of trauma can persist and be triggered by apparently minor things.

Finally, consider the child's current behavior. A child who is in the midst of a flashback, who is acutely agitated, or who is dissociating is not going to be safe to go about his day. A child in this condition needs a quick evaluation to determine whether you can help him stabilize onsite or whether more help is needed.

Onsite Stabilization

Even if you involve CPS or the police, you—in this moment and in the future—play a key role in ensuring the child's ongoing safety. Unfortunately, CPS involvement does not preclude a child's being hurt again. If you can show the child in this instance that you are there to listen, understand, empathize, and help him, he is more likely to come to you should someone hurt him again in the future. As adults, we often assume that children want us to fix the thing that is scaring or upsetting them, and of course when a child is being hurt we want to do just this. But often kids want an adult to listen and truly understand what they are going through, even more than they want it fixed. The role of a police investigator or child protection specialist is to find facts and make determinations, not to empathize with the child (though often these professionals can be highly empathic). If you can listen calmly, understand the child's perspective, empathize about how difficult and complicated his situation is, and validate his experience and his anxieties about the future, this can be a profoundly important intervention.

Catch the Warning Signs

As described in this chapter, many kids who are being abused or who have been through trauma will show it in their behaviors, not their words. Any time a child or teen who has previously been generally successful at school and with social interactions suddenly stops doing well, this should raise a red flag for concern—either for trauma, some other major stress (like bullying or problems at home), or the onset of mental illness. Children and teens will be loathe to talk about any one of these, so how you ask is important. Kids who have been abused or traumatized often feel ashamed and guilty already, so they can be vulnerable to feeling like an adult is saying "What's wrong with you," even if that is not what the adult means. Take a nonjudgmental stance and describe the changes that you have seen, and ask if there has been anything going on that has been bothering them or making things difficult. A traumatized child or teen is much more likely to respond to an adult asking "What happened to you?" rather than "What's wrong with you?" or "You better shape up." Kids often feel better if you can normalize their experience by saying things like "Often I've found when a kid's grades start dropping, it's because something is bothering them and making it hard for them to focus" or "A lot of kids I've seen who have been using weed, use it to get rid of painful feelings or memories." Even if they shrug you off, you are showing that you understand, and they are much more likely to come back and open up later.

Certain groups of kids are at generally increased risk of trauma or abuse, so a sudden change in their behavior should be of particular concern. Children with physical or intellectual disabilities, including kids with autism spectrum disorder, may be targeted because they are vulnerable and less likely to speak up. Children with ADHD or behavior problems are more likely to be abused, perhaps because of their impulsivity and tendency to misbehave. Children in foster care have often been abused, and even if no one has hit them or sexually abused them, being removed from a parent for whatever reason is traumatizing for a child (and even for an adolescent, though they are less likely to admit it). And families under strain can make kids vulnerable to abuse. If you know a family is having serious financial problems, is undergoing a contentious divorce, has just moved into a homeless shelter, or has a caregiver with a major medical illness (particularly if lots of different people are suddenly taking care of the kids), those kids may, in particular, need support and someone watching out for them.

If you know a child has been abused or otherwise traumatized, catching the warning signs becomes about identifying the trauma reminders and triggers that set a child off. Often if a child has been traumatized, their parent is so upset and distressed by what has happened that he or she cannot step back and be an objective observer of triggers for posttraumatic stress symptoms. School staff, therapists, and pediatricians can play a key role in understanding the child's perspective, identifying triggers, and helping parents and caregivers do the same.

Listen and Empathize

As noted at the opening to this section, while your first impulse when you discover a child has been traumatized is to immediately jump into problem-solving mode, take a step back. Children and teens are very attuned to our emotions, and if you get upset or angry or jump to action, this can make them feel more stressed and upset. Most children who have been traumatized want someone first to just listen. Do not push them to tell you all the details, in case they are not ready. Empathize with and validate their experience: "That sounds really scary and hard, and I bet it's hard to talk about. You are being very brave to share this with me, and if it feels like too much to talk about it just let me know and we'll take a break." Ask how they feel, and if they are sad or angry or numb or afraid, try to understand why. If they are able to identify their emotions and their fears, reflect back what they have said ("What I understand from what you have said is that you are afraid how your mom will react, is that right?") and validate their concerns.

If it is a child whose trauma history you already know, and you are intervening now because he had a meltdown or sudden flare of symptoms, the process is similar. Remind the child that you understand why he has these meltdowns: "I know that after what happened with your mom, lots of things can bring back scary memories and bad thoughts. But you know you're safe here and we can figure this out together." Help the child to reflect on what might have been the trigger, and share your observations or those of other staff in a neutral and nonjudgmental way to help fill in the details.

Collaborate to Find Solutions

When a child or teen has revealed a trauma or experience of abuse to you, it is critical that you be honest and transparent about the next steps you plan to take. First, talk with the child about how to make sure he is safe going forward. Who will be picking the child up from school, where will he be staying, will he come back tomorrow, and does he feel safe at each of these steps? If you need to notify the child's parents, the police, or CPS, tell them why and what will happen. Often children and teens have unrealistic fears or misconceptions (e.g., "They'll send me away forever," "They'll put me in jail") that you can remedy, and sometimes their concerns are very valid (e.g., "My mom will be disappointed in me," "My dad's going to kill him"). Hear those concerns and work with the child or teen to find a solution that everyone can feel comfortable with. Even if you have to make a decision (like to notify parents or CPS) that the child is unhappy with, validate his frustration or fear and explain why you must do it anyway.

When working to address posttraumatic stress symptoms or behaviors, you should again take a collaborative stance with the child. There may be trauma reminders you can work together to avoid, or there may be triggers that are unavoidable for which you can help the child develop a plan to cope in advance. For example, sometimes having a "5-minute pass" (a paper pass the student can hold up to get a 5-minute break at the guidance office) can be useful for children who often get triggered during class. Or for an adolescent who has been assaulted, think about a friend who can walk her home on a different route, to avoid the street where the assault occurred, or a strategy that the adolescent can use, like deep relaxation breathing, to manage the stress of having to face her assailant in court. Having been through a traumatic experience does not relieve a child of all responsibilities—we still expect him or her to go to school, come home on time, not use drugs, and so forth—but acknowledge that those things can be difficult and think proactively about how to address them.

Learning From the Crisis

The effects of trauma and abuse can be long-lasting, so it is important to show the child that you are in it with them for the long haul. Talk about the types of difficulties kids can have after a traumatic event (such as the changes in thoughts and feelings described earlier, as well as symptoms like anxiety, depression, and nightmares), and think together about how you might address them if they come up. Help the child to develop a safety plan in which the child identifies the things that act as triggers, the early warning signs that he is having a flashback or other sudden symptom, and what he and others around them can do to help in that moment. Work with the child's family and any therapists or other mental health practitioners who are connected with the child to make sure everyone is on the same page. Often school staff, pediatricians, and others who are close to a child assume that the therapist is aware of the child's trauma history, but the therapist may have no idea or may only know part of the story.

When to Get Help

One of the most difficult decisions when faced with a child's report of abuse or neglect is whether to report to CPS. Many of us who work with children are "mandated reporters"–pediatricians, nurses, teachers, social workers, therapists, child care providers, law enforcement officers, employees, and even volunteers at day care centers or summer camps. Being a mandated reporter means we must call CPS if we have reason to believe a child is being abused or neglected. Often the state reporting hotline provides a consultative service, so if you are not sure whether it is something you should report, you can call and ask and the trained staff on the other end will advise you.

If you suspect a child has been physically or sexually abused, particularly if it has happened recently, you should send the child to the emergency room. The child may have injuries or exposures to sexually transmitted disease that need treatment, or she may need to have a rape kit exam or an examination by a specialist in child abuse pediatrics. Even if the child denies any current physical symptoms, if there has been abuse within the past days or weeks, an emergency evaluation is indicated.

If you are working with a child who has been traumatized in the past but is experiencing acutely dangerous psychiatric symptoms, an emergency evaluation is also needed. If a child is experiencing suicidal thoughts, has been violent and aggressive, or is engaging in dangerous self-harm, he may need to be hospitalized, or at the very least seen quickly by a child psychiatrist, who can assess the level of acute risk and get help for the child.

Finally, it is important to acknowledge the help that you and your team may need after hearing about the abuse or neglect of a child whom you care about. It can be incredibly painful and upsetting to learn that a child whom you work with has been abused or neglected, and many adults in this situation can experience symptoms of vicarious traumatization. These symptoms can include anxiety, depression, nightmares, feelings of guilt or anger or responsibility, difficulty concentrating, and urges to drink or use drugs as a distraction. The child needs you around to help her, so it is as important that you take care of yourself as you take care of her. Spending time with your own loved ones and friends, taking time for relaxation and exercise, and even talking about your feelings with colleagues or a therapist (while protecting the child's confidentiality, of course) can help to reduce your emotional burden and ensure you can be there for the child when she needs you.

References

American Academy of Pediatrics: Helping Foster and Adoptive Families Cope With Trauma: A Guide for Pediatricians. Elk Grove, IL, American Academy of Pediatrics, 2013. Available at: www.aap.org/traumaguide. Accessed April 5, 2014.

American Psychiatric Association: Diagnostic and Statistical Manual of Mental Disorders, 5th Edition. Arlington, VA, American Psychiatric Association, 2013

Bensley LS, Spieker SJ, Van Eenwyk J, et al. Self-reported abuse history and adolescent problem behaviors, II: alcohol and drug use. J Adolesc Health 24:173–180, 1999

Costello EJ, Erkanli A, Fairbank JA, et al: The prevalence of potentially traumatic events in childhood and adolescence. J Traumatic Stress 15(2):99–112, 2002

Flaherty EG, Stirling J, Committee on Child Abuse and Neglect: The pediatrician's role in child maltreatment prevention. Pediatrics 126(833):2010–2087, 2010

Gerson R, Rappaport N: Traumatic stress and posttraumatic stress disorder in youth: recent research findings on clinical impact, assessment, and treatment. J Adolesc Health 52(2):137–143, 2013

U.S. Department of Health and Human Services: Child Maltreatment. Washington, DC, U.S. Department of Health and Human Services, Administration for Children and Families, Children's Bureau, 2010. Available at: http://www.acf.hhs.gov/programs/cb/research-data-technology/statistics-research/child-maltreatment. Accessed April 10, 2014.

Further Readings

Lanius R, Vermetten E, Pain C (eds): The Impact of Early Life Trauma on Health and Disease: The Hidden Epidemic. Cambridge, UK, Cambridge University Press, 2010

Minahan J, Rappaport N: The Behavior Code: A Practical Guide to Understanding and Teaching the Most Challenging Students. Cambridge, MA, Harvard Education Press, 2012

Online Resources for Working With Traumatized Children

Preventing Child Abuse and Neglect

American Academy of Pediatrics: http://www2.aap.org/sections/childabuseneglect/resources.cfm

Online Trainings in Therapy for Childhood Trauma

Medical University of South Carolina: http://tfcbt.musc.edu

Handouts for Children and Families About Coping With Trauma

American Academy of Pediatrics: http://www.aap.org/en-us/advocacy-and-policy/aap-health-initiatives/Medical-Home-for-Children-and-Adolescents-Exposed-to-Violence/Pages/Tools-for-Communities-Families-Parents-and-Kids.aspx

Catch the Warning Signs

1. Identify kids at risk for abuse and maltreatment (kids with physical or intellectual disability, with emotional or behavioral problems, living in foster care, living in poverty, living in dangerous or violent communities).
2. Watch for red flags of abuse and trauma, both physical (unexplained bruises, injuries, or burns; poor hygiene or nutrition; unmet medical needs) and behavioral (sudden changes or symptoms such as hyperactivity, aggression, withdrawal, self-injurious behavior, or truancy).

If You're Working With a Traumatized Child Who Is Upset:

1. Reflect, empathize, and validate the child's feelings and emotions.
2. Try to understand what upset the child, and to identify triggers or trauma reminders.
3. Ask the child what is wrong, what she is feeling, and what she needs.
4. Reflect back what she has told you to make sure you understand, and validate her concerns.

If You Suspect a Child Is Being Abused:

1. Ensure the child is safe.
2. Talk with your supervisor about whether you should notify the child's parents and whether you should notify police.
3. Contact Child Protective Services.
4. If the child is severely agitated, having acute PTSD symptoms, or is having suicidal or homicidal thoughts, refer to the Emergency Room.

De-escalation: Collaborate for Solutions

1. Be honest and transparent about the steps you are going to take (including if you need to call the police or Child Protective Services).
2. Understand and validate the child's concerns.
3. Work with the child to identify triggers, and problem solve together about how to deal with them.

Refer to the Emergency Room if:

1. The child has just reported having been abused and needs a physical and psychological examination.
2. The child expresses suicidal or homicidal thoughts, is severely agitated, or is dissociating.

De-escalation: Learn From the Crisis

1. Help the child to make a plan to cope with trauma triggers that arise in the future.
2. Help the family identify and remove trauma triggers in the environment.
3. Refer for outpatient treatment if you see signs of depression, PTSD, sleep problems, or other psychiatric disorders.

Managing a traumatized child in crisis.

CHAPTER 7

Risky Behaviors

Charles J. Glawe, M.D.

Television, movies, and news might lead you to believe that every teenager is skipping school, driving around in fast cars, and experimenting with drugs, alcohol, and sex. It is certainly true that adolescence is a time of transition during which children are growing into adulthood, testing their boundaries, and learning (we hope) from their mistakes. But typically, a teenager learns to navigate the experience of becoming an adult much like a child might learn to navigate a swimming pool. Most start out wading in the shallow end of the pool, learning the basics of how to navigate around, and relying on the nearest adult to teach them how to keep their head above water.

It is concerning, therefore, when we see a teenager begin to dive off into the deep end of the proverbial pool. Adolescence is a time of exploration and testing boundaries, but dangerous, risky behaviors are not the norm. Risky and potentially dangerous behaviors can be a sign of possible social or family problems, poor supervision, or more serious mental illness. School truancy, running away, experimentation with drugs, gang involvement, and risky sexual behaviors can derail and even threaten the life of an adolescent who does not yet have the ability to fully cope with adult issues and decisions. It is imperative that the warning signs of risky behaviors be recognized and appropriately addressed to prevent the teenager from drowning in bad decisions.

Case Presentation

Lisa is a 15-year-old freshman in high school. Up until recently, Lisa has been a good student, well liked by her teachers and classmates, with many friends. Over the last several months, however, Lisa has been missing more and more days of school, beginning with one day every couple of weeks and increasing to 2–3 days every week. Her grades have gradually slipped from an A average to barely passing, and she has consistently failed to turn in assignments. Teachers report that Lisa appears sullen, irritable, and withdrawn at times during the day. Two weeks ago she was caught outside on school property smoking cigarettes with a classmate, and she was briefly suspended.

Today Lisa has not shown up to school again, and the school has not been notified by a parent. An administrator calls home and receives a report that Lisa's mother does not know where she is. Lisa reportedly did not come home after school the previous night, and the family has not heard anything from her since she left for school the previous morning. Calls to friends and other contacts have come up empty, and Lisa's mother is worried. She notes that Lisa has threatened to run away several times in the last month after arguments about her curfew, but has never been missing overnight without contacting her family. After hanging up with the school, Lisa's mother calls police.

Understanding the Crisis

While any behavior that is potentially limiting or dangerous to an adolescent should be identified and consideration taken as to its potential impact on his or her ability to function, there are a number of behaviors and problems that are commonly seen in adolescents who are at risk for more serious mental illness.

Truancy

As noted in our case example, truancy can often be an early warning sign in children of more serious problems. It is frequently missed or overlooked, but it can be a behavior common to many mental illnesses from anxiety disorders and depression, to behavioral disorders such as oppositional defiant disorder (ODD) and conduct disorder as well as substance abuse. Its impact is also significant both for what the adolescent is missing (her education and important social/developmental experiences) and for what she is doing instead of being in school (being unsupervised and engaging in other risky behaviors). Increasing or frequent truancy should be addressed early to help prevent academic difficulty and other consequences.

Runaway Behavior

While it is not uncommon for children to express a desire to live on their own or frustration with parent rules, it is another thing entirely for a child to act on these thoughts and run away from home. Leaving the supervision of parents or guardians puts the adolescent in a position of having to care for his needs himself, which is a significant responsibility for an adult, let alone a teenager, who usually does not have the means or emotional maturity to live on his own. If an adolescent chooses this over his home, it is likely that either the situation at home is so unbearable that he can no longer tolerate it, or the adolescent has internal problems that keep him from recognizing the limitations on his abilities. Either or both are cause for concern.

Substance Use

Our case example for this chapter makes mention of possible tobacco use in a teen, and this should not be overlooked. Not only is tobacco use itself a risk factor for numerous medical problems, it is frequently found to be more prevalent in adolescents and adults with a variety of mental illnesses (Smith et al. 2014). It should also prompt questioning on use of other substances, including alcohol, marijuana, and other drugs.

Risky Sexual Behavior

Learning to navigate relationships and explore sexuality is an important developmental task for adolescents. The consequences of impulsive or risky behaviors can include unintended pregnancies, sexually transmitted infections, and even sexual exploitation in the form of underage prostitution. Various mental illnesses can contribute to teens engaging in more impulsive and risky sexual practices, and a recognition of these behaviors is important in minimizing long-term consequences and keeping adolescents safe.

Identifying Kids at Risk

The first step in dealing with risky behaviors in adolescents is recognizing that the behavior is outside of normal adolescent behavior and potentially an indication of a more serious problem. One way to determine whether the behavior is indicative of a more serious problem is by considering how the average teenager behaves. Taking Lisa's case as an example, we might think that missing a day of school on occasion due to an illness, a doctor's appointment, or a major life event would be a common occurrence, on average, for any teenager. Missing 2–3 days a week, on the other hand, may seem beyond what the average adolescent experiences and could be cause for concern.

This approach can be helpful for behavior in which the average is well known and the behavior in question is well outside of what is considered normal. The problem with comparing a given behavior with the average is that there is the risk of missing behaviors that are misperceived as being more common than they actually are. For example, if one watches the average teenage television drama, it might be assumed that nearly every adolescent has had sex with multiple partners by the time they are 16 years old. While sexual activity is not uncommon in teenagers, one would be overstating how common it is if this was the assumption of the norm. Similarly, a schoolteacher working in a special education classroom for students with behavioral problems is going to have a different perception of the average truancy rate for an adolescent when compared with a teacher in a gifted education science class.

Another way in which clinicians identify potential warning-sign behaviors is by considering what impact the behavior is having on the adolescent's ability to function. Any behavior that has an adverse impact on an adolescent's social, academic, or family functioning is a cause for concern. Identifying potentially risky and problematic behaviors in this way places more of the focus on the individual and her functioning and less on comparing her with other adolescents. This approach has the advantage of taking into account the situation that a particular individual is in and tailoring the response to that person.

A related warning sign that many child mental health practitioners use to identify potentially problematic behaviors that may be overlying more serious mental illness is any change in an individual's behavior or level of functioning. Such change is clearly illustrated in our previous example, as Lisa is noted to previously have been a student with an A average who appears to have been functioning relatively well with teachers and socially with friends. Over time, Lisa's functioning appears to have deteriorated, particularly with regard to her academic functioning, which has declined significantly because of her truancy and difficulty completing assignments. This should be a warning sign that something is adversely affecting Lisa's ability to attend school and function appropriately.

It should be noted in this example that the change in Lisa's functioning happens relatively gradually over a period of several months. Gradual changes can be more difficult to identify than abrupt changes in behavior. The child who is attending school regularly and then suddenly stops coming altogether is easier to identify than the child who gradually decreases his attendance, because we more easily become accustomed to small changes over a longer period of time than we do to large changes over a shorter period of time.

Clinicians conceptualize factors that contribute to the development of problematic behaviors and mental illness by considering the biological, psychological, and social influences in a child's life. A number of characteristics contribute to the development of risky behaviors in adolescents.

Impulsivity

Adequate impulse control enables individuals to control their initial reaction to a situation in favor of reasoning out the most advantageous result and adjusting their behavior accordingly. Individuals with poor impulse control have a tendency to react before they have thought out the consequences of a situation. Adolescence is, under normal circumstances, a period in which individuals are more prone to impulsiveness and less able to think through the consequences of their actions (Dreyfuss et al. 2014). There are various disorders, however, that can make an adolescent even more prone to acting impulsively, such as attention-deficit/hyperactivity disorder (ADHD), certain anxiety disorders, and mania in a teen with bipolar disorder. Poor impulse control can be a difficult characteristic to treat but often improves with age and experience.

Grandiosity

The term *grandiosity* refers to some individuals' tendency to think they are more capable with regard to a certain trait or in a given situation and to minimize the potential likelihood or impact of consequences of a given behavior. The ancient Greek concept of hubris or the idea of an over-inflated ego might be thought of as similar concepts. As with impulsivity, adolescents are prone, even in normal development, to more grandiose thinking than is typical of adults. The concept of teenagers believing they are "invincible" can lead them to minimize the possible negative impacts of risky behaviors and engage in actions that an older, experienced adult would not even consider undertaking (Calvete 2008).

Differential Diagnosis

The list of mental health diagnoses that can contribute to risky behaviors in adolescents is broad. Knowledge of various mental illnesses and how they contribute to risky behaviors can help you to know when to refer a child or adolescent for a psychiatric evaluation, as well as how to manage symptoms and treatment in everyday life once a diagnosis has been established.

Attention-Deficit/Hyperactivity Disorder

The symptoms of ADHD include difficulty with maintaining attention, hyperactivity, and impulsivity. Any of these symptoms can contribute in significant ways to children and adolescents engaging in more risky behaviors. Impulsivity, however, is of particular concern, as it does, by definition, impair an adolescent's ability to reason through decisions on how to act. The adolescent with ADHD may be more susceptible to the effects of peer pressure, or may be more likely to engage in behavior without considering the consequences. It is not uncommon for children and adolescents with ADHD to engage in risky behavior on impulse and later to regret their behavior, having not adequately thought through what they were doing in the first place.

Disruptive Behavior Disorders

Disruptive behavior disorders encompass both ODD and conduct disorder and are highly associated with a number of risky behaviors. Disruptive behavior disorders also commonly co-occur with other types of mental health disorders such as ADHD, various mood disorders, and a history of previous trauma or neglect. (Roy et al. 2014).

ODD is characterized by a lack of regard for rules and authority figures. Children with ODD may often get along relatively well with peers and in peer social situations, but they have a difficult time following rules or following the directions of an adult or person of authority. Given that many risky behaviors are themselves in opposition to societal rules or laws, it should come as no surprise that a child with ODD would be predisposed to a number of risky behaviors.

Of even greater concern is a diagnosis of conduct disorder, which is characterized by repeated patterns of behavior that violate societal rules, laws, or the rights of others. Adolescents with conduct disorder may engage in acts of aggression, theft, vandalism, and serious rules violations that make them particularly susceptible to high-risk behaviors. Many risky behaviors, including significant truancy, running away from home, dangerous sexual activities, and activities related to gang involvement, are themselves considered diagnostic criteria for conduct disorder.

Mood Disorders, Including Depression and Bipolar Disorder

Mood disorders in children and adolescents can often manifest differently than in adults and can contribute to risk-taking behaviors. In adults, depression is often notable for characteristic sad mood, social isolation, decreased energy, poor sleep, and difficulty with concentration and the ability to complete tasks. These symptoms can be noted in children and adolescents as well, though teens are also likely to appear irritable, agitated, and sometimes oppositional in response to depression (Whelan et al. 2013). In fact, a depressed child or adolescent may not even describe himself as depressed or sad, but may instead appear angry and even act out his depression by engaging in behaviors that can, at times, be dangerous. It is particularly important to consider depression in a youth exhibiting a new onset of risky behaviors, because the behaviors may be an indication of the onset of a depressive episode, and the depression can easily be overlooked by those assuming that someone who is depressed will appear sad.

Youths with bipolar disorder can also have periods of depression that are characterized by irritability, agitation, and oppositional behaviors without clear evidence of sadness. In addition, they will exhibit periods of mania which can also predispose them to risky behaviors. Mania is characterized by symptoms that are sometimes thought of as the opposite of depression, including an elevated mood, increased energy, decreased need for sleep, increased interest in sexual activity, impulsive behaviors, and at times even grandiose and delusional thinking. Adolescents with mania can be prone to risky behaviors due to a combination of these factors. A grandiose sense of self can lead those with mania to believe that they are less likely to experience possible consequences of high-risk behaviors, and can even give them a sense of invincibility. The increased energy and elevated mood of adolescents with mania can also lead them to minimize the consequences of risky behaviors. As has already been noted, impulsivity can result in adolescents engaging in behaviors before they have even considered what the consequences might be. Mania has a high correlation with risky behaviors and should be a clear reason for seeking mental health treatment of adolescents who are at risk.

Anxiety and Anxiety Disorders

Anxiety can be a powerful motivator in children and adolescents and results in avoidance of things that are important in development. Anxiety is commonly seen in cases of significant truancy from school and might very easily be misinterpreted as oppositional or conduct-disordered behavior (Egger et al. 2004). In reality, an adolescent may develop significant anxiety about schoolwork related to poor performance, a learning disorder, or difficulty with a particular subject. She may also develop anxiety related to social situations, such as those involving school bullying, separation anxiety, or social anxiety. Anxiety in these situations can lead to the student's skipping school or leaving school when confronted with an anxiety-producing situation in an attempt to avoid the anxiety she is experiencing. In addition, adolescents with significant anxiety can be prone to substance abuse as a way of alleviating or coping with the anxiety they experience (Adams et al. 2013).

Special attention should also be given to adolescents who have experienced physical, emotional, or sexual trauma, including physical abuse, neglect, sexual assault, significant medical illness, or a disaster or major accident. Many children and adolescents experiencing significant trauma can develop posttraumatic stress disorder. Even those without this diagnosis can be significantly affected by a traumatic event. Trauma can produce significant anxiety and hyperarousal leading to avoidance of places, people, or events that remind those affected of their previous trauma. Significant anxiety can, as previously noted, lead to significant substance use as a way of coping with the trauma. Many traumatized children and adolescents may act out or become oppositional to authority as another way of coping with the complex feelings that a traumatic event can produce. Oppositional behavior and difficulty trusting authority can particularly be a problem when the trauma was caused by a parent or guardian, either directly through physical, emotional, or sexual abuse or less directly through negligence or neglect. Children and adolescents may also experience significant guilt related to a traumatic experience, either when they believe they are somehow to blame for the experience or, in some cases, when they have survived an event in which others have died or been seriously hurt. Guilt can, in some cases, result in adolescents continuing to engage in dangerous and harmful behaviors as a way to alleviate the guilt they may feel. Finally, some adolescents who have experienced trauma may appear to put themselves into situations that may reproduce the trauma they have previously experienced. Although this may appear contrary to what one might expect, the ability to reexperience and tolerate further trauma as a way of gaining some measure of control can be a powerful motivator. Adolescents exhibiting these types of reactions to previous traumatic experiences require appropriate mental health treatment to help them learn to cope with the significant, sometimes conflicted, feelings that prior trauma can produce.

Identifying Immediate Triggers

In addition to assessing chronic factors, such as mental illness, that can lead a teen to engage in risky behaviors, often there is a series of events that leads them in this one moment to run away, skip school, or start to go on a drinking binge. It is important to pay attention to **changes in the child's mood** and other behaviors, since as noted earlier, an episode of depression or mania or a worsening of anxiety symptoms might trigger risky behaviors. **Environmental changes** can also contribute. If the parent is out of the home more in the evening visiting an ill grandparent in the hospital, a child might have more of an opportunity for drinking or partying, or may be acting out due to anger at the parent for not being home or worry about the ill grandparent. Divorce or a parent starting a new romantic relationship is also often a trigger for more frequent risky behaviors, as it changes the parent's ability to supervise the child and often triggers strong emotions in the child as well. Even when there are not major changes happening at home, an argument with parents–or even fear of an argument or punishment (e.g., if an adolescent knows she is failing a class and fears her parents' disapproval)–is often the immediate trigger for running away or for substance use. Getting at these immediate triggers often requires **taking the child's perspective,** which can be difficult when you are worried that the child is putting herself in danger. But identifying these immediate triggers can help you to know when parents, teachers, and others should be on "high alert" in the future to prevent the child's acting out again.

Risk Assessment

Risk assessment is important in the evaluation of children with risky behaviors both in the acute management of a crisis and in determining when and how to intervene before high-risk behaviors begin to put the adolescent at imminent risk (Table 7–1). For a child engaging in risky behaviors, the first step is to make certain that the adolescent is not in a situation that is immediately dangerous to his safety. First consider the environment the child is currently in. Who is the child with, and is he being monitored by a trusted adult? If the child is with an adult who can safely monitor his behavior, the risk is not as acute as it is for a child who is either not currently under adult supervision or under supervision that is in some way inadequate. Peers can significantly influence children, and children who are with others who are also engaging in high-risk behaviors are also at increased risk. Does the environment the child is in represent an imminent danger to him? A child at school or with capable parents at home is at less risk than a child who is out with friends on the street. A child who is missing is at significant risk, because his current environment cannot be evaluated and he has no adequate supervision.

The next thing to consider in acute management is the behavior in which the child is currently engaging. Children with a history of high-risk

TABLE 7–1. Risk factors for risk-taking behaviors

Environmental factors	Peers engaging in risky behaviors
	Lack of parental/adult supervision
	Alcohol or prescription medications available in the home
Child factors	Impulsivity
	Grandiosity
Psychiatric illness	Attention-deficit/hyperactivity disorder
	Disruptive behavior disorders
	Mood disorders (depression, bipolar disorder)
	Anxiety disorders
	Posttraumatic stress disorder
Immediate triggers	Problems at school
	Conflict or changes at home

behaviors are at the highest risk when they are actively engaged in those behaviors. A child who has a history of substance abuse, for example, is at the most vulnerable when she is intoxicated. A child with a history of truancy is at highest risk when he has skipped school and is out on the street unsupervised. The most acute need for intervention in an emergency situation is when the child either is actively engaged in the behavior or has indicated that she will be engaged in the behavior in the near future.

In our previous example of school truancy, Lisa was noted to have been missing overnight, and neither her friends nor her family were aware of where she currently was at the time that the school called home to notify them of her absence. Lisa's functioning had been declining over the past several months, which would be concerning itself with regard to her risk assessment. Disappearing overnight, however, is even more uncharacteristic of her typical behavior and cause for concern. The immediate goal in a situation in which a child is in immediate danger is to remove them from the immediate situation. In this case, finding Lisa and returning her to her family is the immediate response.

Evaluating an adolescent's risk when he or she is not immediately involved in a risky behavior or in imminent danger is a more complex task. Past behavior is the strongest predictor of future behavior, and people who have previously engaged in activities that may be dangerous to their well-being are more likely to engage in these behaviors in the future. In Lisa's example, her worsening school attendance, academic performance, and tobacco use predict future poor attendance, academic performance, and tobacco use if there is no intervention designed to change these behaviors and treat any pathology contributing to them. Thus, these behaviors could serve as a marker for potential risk in the future.

Onsite Stabilization

In situations that involve the potential for imminent harm to the adolescent, the first step is to get the teen out of immediate danger. An adolescent who has not shown up to school must be found or a parent notified that he is missing. A teen who is intoxicated should be taken out of harm's way and put under proper adult supervision. A child who is being sexually exploited must have her case reported to the appropriate state authority for children's services. The first step in any situation, regardless of the behavior in question, must be to ensure the adolescent's immediate safety and proper supervision.

Once any imminent danger is addressed, more information needs to be obtained. Potential risky behaviors that may eventually put an adolescent in harm's way, or be detrimental to her emotional, academic, or social development, need to be identified and a proper risk assessment made. In many cases, a single episode of truancy or cigarette smoking can be easily addressed with a brief discussion with the teen, appropriate disciplinary action, and notification of a parent or guardian. Patterns of behavior, however, need to be addressed, and possible causes or other risk factors need to be identified to determine the proper course of action. In particular, any evidence of mental illness, such as depression, mania, anxiety, reactions to abusive situations, and substance use, and any other indication of possible difficulty in functioning should be identified so that referral to an appropriate mental health professional can be considered.

Catch the Warning Signs

When one is trying to address risky behaviors, it is crucial to look at potential triggers and risk factors in all of the environments where a child spends time. For a teacher or other school official, it is vital to obtain as much information as is practical about the home environment. Are there significant changes that are happening at home, such as the illness of a family member, or a divorce? These stressors can have a significant impact on how an adolescent functions and might become apparent in the school environment. How parents have already tried to deal with problem behaviors can also be helpful information when determining how to help. Parents very frequently use punishment as a means of disciplining children who engage in problematic behaviors. Although this can be helpful in some cases, it can also promote power struggles between adolescents and parents. Once this pattern is established and the teen stops responding to punishment, it can be a difficult cycle to correct.

Similarly, it is important for parents to pay close attention to what adolescents are coping with in a school environment. A teenager who is truant may, in fact, be avoiding school because of poor performance due to a learning disorder. An adolescent who is being bullied at school or feels physically threatened often may not feel comfortable talking about the situation with an adult and can act out her frustration in other ways. Clear, honest, and frequent communication between parents and educators can help identify important missing information that may shed light on an otherwise confusing pattern of problematic behavior.

Listen and Empathize

It can be difficult talking to adolescents about risky behaviors. For one thing, the topics can be difficult ones for an adult in a position of authority or caregiving to bring up with an adolescent. You might think that an adolescent would not want to talk to an adult about topics like drugs, sex, or difficulty in school, but the reality is often very different from what adults might expect. It is true that teenagers often do not voluntarily offer information about topics like these to adults, but it is also true that many adolescents are confused and conflicted about these issues and may appreciate having an adult they can trust to speak with about them. The key in speaking with adolescents about difficult topics is finding a balance between setting appropriate limits with them and providing a nonjudgmental ear for them and a source of support. Concern for their safety and empathy for the difficult transition that adolescence often is can be helpful in gaining trust and in ensuring that they get whatever help and assistance that they need.

Adults sometimes worry about causing more harm than good in bringing up difficult topics with adolescents, particularly topics like sex, drug use, or even thoughts of depression or suicide. It is important to realize that simply asking an adolescent if she is sexually active will not make her more likely to engage in sexual activity. Neither will asking a teenager if she is depressed or suicidal cause her to want to kill herself. In fact, it is much more likely that by having the opportunity to talk about feeling depressed, a teen will be less likely to kill herself than if she had no one to speak with about how she was feeling. Talking about difficult subjects gives caregivers the opportunity to address whatever concerns and potential problems an adolescent has, and this in turn can help prevent these problems from becoming worse.

Once it is determined that an adolescent is engaging in a risky behavior, as much detail as possible should be obtained. If a teenager is drinking alcohol, how much alcohol? What type of alcohol? When did she start drinking? How often does she drink? Where does she get her alcohol? Has she ever gotten drunk? Has her drinking caused her to get into trouble? Why does she drink? Is it a social function, or does she drink to alleviate stress she has at home or school? The more information that can be obtained, the more appropriate a response can be formulated.

Collaborate to Find Solutions

Oftentimes, noncomplex issues can be addressed with appropriate consequences for inappropriate behavior and education. Again, teaching teenagers about safe sex practices or the consequences of drug use does not make them more likely to engage in these behaviors. It gives them the tools they need to make informed and safe decisions about their behaviors. The effectiveness of positive reinforcement in shaping behavior should also not be overlooked. Praise and rewards can be just as important, if not more so, than punishment. For example, punishing a child for skipping school may not end the truancy problem, but an intervention by a teacher or counselor may lead to the child attending school more regularly. Many common problems with teens can be solved with a simple, frank conversation and a little support and attention.

Learning From the Crisis

Many adolescents, when confronted in an empathic, nonjudgmental way about their risky behaviors, will sheepishly acknowledge the validity of the adults' concerns and accept more supervision and support. Others will admit that their behavior has been a cry for help. In these cases, working to address the underlying factors that led to the risky behaviors will often be sufficient to stop the behavior. If the child refuses to acknowledge the dangerousness of his or her behaviors and is not motivated to change, it may be necessary to involve law enforcement or Child Protective Services. See Chapter 8, "Clinical and Forensic Psychological Issues With At-Risk Youths and Juvenile Delinquents," for information about these programs.

When to Get Help

Many minor behavioral problems can be dealt with through information gathering, involvement of parents, education, and support. In situations involving more serious risky behaviors or signs of possible mental illness, further support may be needed.

Truancy becomes a problem that may need further intervention when it becomes frequent enough to impact a child's education or safety and when typical interventions to address it have been ineffective. If a teen continues to be truant after clear limit setting, appropriate consequences, and an attempt to identify any obvious source of stress at school, it is likely time to seek additional help. Of particular concern are adolescents who refuse to go to school altogether. The longer a child refuses to go to school, the more difficult it becomes to help her become reintegrated into her educational and social environment at school. In the case of school truancy, referral to an appropriate mental health professional for evaluation is usually enough to provide some understanding of what may be contributing to the problem and how to solve it. In cases where a teen refuses to go to see a professional, or if he completely refuses to leave the home, it may be helpful for the parent to go to speak with the therapist first to provide information and get help in strategies for getting the adolescent to go to the appointment. If this is not effective, there are situations in which bringing a team or individual therapist to the home to conduct an interview may be appropriate. Rarely will an adolescent need to be forcibly removed or taken to an emergency room (ER). This intervention should be reserved for situations in which the teen will not cooperate and the behavior she is engaging in is imminently dangerous to her health or safety.

Problematic substance use can range in dangerousness from regular cigarette or alcohol use that places the long-term health of an adolescent at risk, to very serious addiction and dependence on heroin, cocaine, crystal meth, and other dangerous substances. For use that is less imminently dangerous but still concerning for long-term health risks, education and clear limit setting can be helpful. Often the place to start may be the teenager's regular doctor or pediatrician. Pediatricians and family doctors are well equipped to discuss the dangers of long-term drug, alcohol, or tobacco use and can also provide less complex treatments such as smoking cessation programs when they are needed. Adolescents with more significant substance use problems should be referred to a child mental health professional, preferably one who has expertise in child and adolescent substance abuse. Outpatient substance abuse treatment, including counseling, groups, and medication when appropriate, can be very effective in dealing with mild and moderate problematic substance use. In more severe cases of addiction and dependence, inpatient rehabilitation designed for an adolescent population may be needed. As for truancy, ER visits should be reserved for teens who are dangerous with regard to their substance use. Examples might be a teen who is engaged in dangerous behavior while intoxicated, a teen who has overdosed on a drug or is unresponsive, or a teen who is having dangerous withdrawal from alcohol or another drug.

Like problematic substance use, risky sexual behavior should often first be addressed by the adolescent's pediatrician or family doctor. In this case, testing for sexually acquired diseases, proper physical exam, and testing for pregnancy in girls is important even before the behavior itself is examined. Once the adolescent's health needs have been properly addressed, a pediatrician or family doctor can provide education on safe sex practices, as well as condoms and birth control options when needed. In cases of recurrent risky sexual behaviors that put an adolescent at risk, a referral to an appropriate mental health professional is needed in addition to the medical exam conducted by the primary physician. Emergency room visits are again appropriate only in cases in which the child's health or safety are in jeopardy. Known unprotected sex with a person with HIV or AIDS, recent physical trauma from sexual practices, or recent rape or sexual assault may be reasons to seek help on an emergency basis.

Of all of the risky behaviors discussed, runaway behavior has the most potential to be dangerous and is most likely to result in the need for professional intervention. As mentioned previously, a teenager who has run away from home is particularly vulnerable because she does not have adequate adult supervision and in most cases does not have the ability to adequately care for herself. Recommendations and state laws vary with regard to filing reports on missing children, but the safest recommendation and the opinion of this writer is that any time a child or adolescent is missing and her whereabouts cannot be determined, law enforcement should be notified. Although it is possible the child may return shortly after expending some anger, she may be in significant danger of being exploited by other adults or engaging in other risky behaviors when not under appropriate adult supervision. The chance of finding a missing child drops significantly the longer she is missing. In situations where a child is repeatedly running away from home, professional intervention is needed. Individual evaluation of the child by a trained mental health professional, and often evaluation of the family and interaction between parents and the child, may be needed to help repair difficult relationships between a frequent runaway and her parents.

In all cases of risky and problematic behaviors, referral to an ER or calling 911 should generally be reserved only for situations that present an imminent danger to the health and well-being of the adolescent involved. Although it may seem that it is better to quickly address even more minor issues and ensure that the adolescent is followed up, a visit to the ER can be time consuming, expensive, and sometimes traumatic and frightening to a teenager who is likely already under a great deal of stress. ERs are designed to triage patients by level of acuity, and psychiatric emergency services are meant to determine whether a patient is dangerous and in need of immediate admission to a psychiatric hospital, or whether the patient is safe and follow up with an outpatient evaluation at a later date is more appropriate. Generally patients with more minor issues are given only the brief emergency evaluation and a referral to follow-up with an outpatient provider. In non-life-threatening situations, this can be more easily accomplished with a simple referral to an appropriate outpatient clinic or private mental health practitioner.

References

Adams ZW, McCart MR, Zajac K, et al: Psychiatric problems and trauma exposure in nondetained delinquent and nondelinquent adolescents. J Clin Child Adolesc Psychol 42(3):323–331, 2013

Calvete E: Justification of violence and grandiosity schemas as predictors of antisocial behavior in adolescents. J Abnorm Child Psychol 36(7):1083–1095, 2008

Dreyfuss M, Caudle K, Drysdale AT, et al: Teens impulsively react rather than retreat from threat. Dev Neurosci May 8, 2014 [Epub ahead of print]

Egger HL, Costello EJ, Angold A: School refusal and psychiatric disorders: a community study. J Am Acad Child Adolesc Psychiatry 42(7):797–807, 2004

Roy A, Oldehinkel AJ, Verhulst FC, et al: Anxiety and disruptive behavior mediate pathways from attention-deficit/hyperactivity disorder to depression. J Clin Psychiatry 75(2):e108–113, 2014

Smith PH, Mazure CM, McKee SA: Smoking and mental illness in the US population. Tob Control April 17, 2014 [Epub ahead of print]

Whelan YM, Stringaris A, Maughan B, Barker ED: Developmental continuity of oppositional defiant disorder subdimensions at ages 8, 10, and 13 and their distinct psychiatric outcomes at age 16 years. J Am Acad Child Adolesc Psychiatry 52(9):961–969, 2013

Identify Adolescents at Risk

1. Know what is typical behavior for an average adolescent.
2. Identify any gradual or abrupt changes in behavior.
3. Address any behaviors that may impair an adolescent's ability to function.

Assess the Level of Risk

1. Is the teen being supervised by a responsible adult?
2. Is the teen in imminent physical danger or medically at risk?
3. Is the child currently engaged in dangerous or risky behavior?

Gather Additional Information

1. Are there any significant changes at home?
2. Are there any significant changes at school?
3. What stressors are affecting the teen's life?
4. What details about the behavior can be identified?

Call for Help or Refer to the Emergency Room if:

1. The teen is missing or in inadequate supervision.
2. The teen is intoxicated or medically ill.
3. The teen is currently engaged in behavior that is an imminent risk.

Talk to the Teen

1. Don't be afraid to approach difficult topics.
2. Set appropriate limits while trying to remain nonjudgmental.
3. Educate teens about safe alternatives to problem behaviors.

Get Help When Needed

1. Make sure to involve parents, family, and schools when needed.
2. Refer to a pediatrician for any needed medical workup or health education.
3. Involve a trained mental health professional when mental illness is suspected or when other interventions have failed.

Addressing high-risk behaviors in adolescents.

CHAPTER 8

Clinical and Forensic Psychological Issues With At-Risk Youths and Juvenile Delinquents

Alessandra D.E. Herbosch, Psy.D.

There are few things more horrifying for a parent than getting a call that their child has been arrested. Children and adolescents can become involved in criminal behaviors for many reasons, but for many youths, unrecognized or untreated mental health problems have put them on a trajectory that ends with the legal system. As many as 70% of youths in the juvenile justice system have a mental illness (Skowyra and Cocozza 2007). Recognizing and treating that mental illness, and understanding the ways that mental illness can make adolescents more likely to commit a crime, can help determine the most appropriate intervention for a child and reduce recidivism rates.

A child or adolescent can become involved with law enforcement in several ways. For example, he may have committed an offense (e.g., gang involvement, drug involvement, assaulted someone); he may have been a victim of a crime (e.g., sexually abused, bullied by peers, forced into prostitution); or he may have become involved with the courts because of environmental and sociocultural issues (e.g., child protection, contentious custody battles, parental legal issues). At times there can be overlap between these situations—for example, when a child is both the victim of a crime and has a criminal history herself. And mental health problems can be at play in any of these scenarios; a psychotic teen may assault a classmate in response to hallucinations telling him to do so; a child may become depressed because of abuse or bullying; and a child may develop posttraumatic stress disorder (PTSD) after witnessing violent arguments between her divorcing parents.

Case Presentation

Adam, age 16, is brought to the emergency room (ER) in police custody after an outburst at school. The school safety officer that accompanies them says Adam had become suddenly enraged at a classmate, screaming and threatening him, and then lunged at the student, grabbed a chair, and swung it at the student's head. Adam threatened to hit anyone else who came toward him. Once school safety officers appeared, Adam was restrained, the police were called, and Adam was brought to the hospital for further evaluation. Adam is still out of control in the ER and attempts to assault both police and hospital staff.

Adam is currently living with his aunt after he reported domestic violence and physical abuse by his parents. Adam was diagnosed with attention-deficit/hyperactivity disorder (ADHD) when he was 8, and since then he has also been diagnosed with PTSD (due to the physical abuse and domestic violence) and conduct disorder (due to truancy, assaulting a teacher at school, threatening classmates, numerous fights at school, and theft and destruction of school property). He was psychiatrically hospitalized on three occasions for past violence with the intent to harm others, and arrested on one occasion for theft. In the ER, Adam's parents were contacted and described a long history of aggressive behaviors and severe temper tantrums. He has assaulted his parents and destroyed things in the house on multiple occasions, and he was expelled from two schools because of violence and truancy. He has run away from home on multiple occasions, comes home drunk, and refuses to see his therapist or psychiatrist. Both parents acknowledged past instances of domestic violence in the home (father has been arrested twice for domestic violence) and admitted that they "disciplined" Adam in order to make him stop his violent outbursts. In addition, Adam's mother struggles with bipolar disorder.

Understanding the Crisis

Adam's case is very complex and has several overlapping components on individual, social, and legal levels. On an individual level, Adam is a teenage boy with a long history of aggression and violent behavior, he has witnessed domestic violence, he has a genetic predisposition to a psychiatric illness, he has been the victim of abuse, he has multiple psychiatric illnesses for which he refuses treatment, and he is abusing alcohol. Psychologically, his ADHD makes him impulsive, and his history of abuse means that he assumes adults will hurt him and often misinterprets things people do as threatening or hostile. From a social perspective, he comes from a chaotic and violent home, with parents who are themselves mentally ill, and now has been removed from the home by Child Protective Services (CPS). Legally, we have an adolescent who is involved with the legal system because of his parents' abusing him, and also he himself has committed two separate types of offenses. First, Adam has committed crimes known as **status offenses.** These are offenses, such as underage drinking, a minor purchasing of cigarettes, running away from home, and truancy, that are only considered as a crime because of the child's *status* as a minor. Adam would also be considered a **juvenile delinquent** because he is under the age of 18 and committed a past crime (e.g., theft), in addition to his status offenses. Remember that while most states have 18 as the age cutoff, some states, such as Connecticut, New York, and North Carolina, consider the cutoff for juvenile delinquency to be age 16, and in some states children as young as 13 may be tried as adults for certain crimes.

The combination of these risk factors has led to Adam's aggressive outburst today. Could this outburst have been prevented, and can future violence and criminality be avoided?

Identifying Kids at Risk

Each year, American schools see more than 800,000 nonfatal violent events within their walls (Robers et al. 2012). School shootings (some of them fatal) have become more common in the past 15 years, with some perpetrators as young as 6 ("Timeline of Worldwide School and Mass Shootings" 2012). Drug use and selling drugs, gang involvement, and prostitution are also sadly not uncommon in our schools and communities. Children and adolescents can also face legal charges and consequences if they engage in cyberbullying, sexting, hacking, or other online activities.

Seventy percent of the two million juveniles arrested each year have a diagnosed mental health disorder, with potentially more having undiagnosed psychiatric illness (Puzzanchera 2009; Skowyra and Cocozza 2007; Teplin et al. 2002; Wasserman et al. 2002). Twenty percent of arrested youths have severe long-term psychological impairments that will continue to affect their functioning into adulthood (Cocozza and Skowyra 2000; Shufelt and Cocozza 2006; Skowyra and Cocozza 2007). Although most children with psychiatric issues will never commit a crime, identifying those young people who do have mental illness and getting them help may prevent their committing a crime or becoming involved in the criminal justice system.

Mental illness is only one risk factor for criminal behavior. We can think about risk factors for criminality as occurring on an *individual* level or on an *environmental* level, including issues in the family. On an **individual** level, adolescents can be at risk for criminal behavior because adolescents are impulsive. Brain development continues until the early 20s, and the parts that develop the most slowly are the areas that allow impulse control, emotional maturity, moral decision making, and the ability to fully comprehend the ramifications of one's actions and consequences. If a child has been exposed to drugs in the prenatal period, or if there are genetic factors that increase their risk for **impulsivity** (such as parental ADHD, bipolar disorder, or aggression/criminality), this risk can be exacerbated. Youths who are using drugs or alcohol will also be even more impulsive, because their thinking and judgment are impaired by the substances. Depending on the cognitive level and capacity for impulse control of a specific child, different interventions will be more or less effective to prevent criminal behaviors. Children and adolescents who have been brought up in violent homes or communities often experience **cognitive distortions** and misinterpret situations or individuals as being hostile. (For example, if a peer bumps into the child accidentally, the child assumes it was on purpose and with malicious intent or "disrespect.") These distortions are often learned, though it is possible that children with PTSD (particularly if it is the result of physical abuse) or disruptive behavior disorders (such as oppositional defiant disorder [ODD] or conduct disorder) might be particularly vulnerable to this due to the neurobiological effects of their illness.

On an **environmental** level, studies have identified six major risk factors: low socioeconomic status, parental criminality, maternal mental illness, severe marital discord between parents, overcrowding in the home or large family size, and a child's placement outside the home—specifically in foster care or residential placement (Rutter 1985). In general, family and parenting factors are a strong influence on the origin of misconduct, aggression, and criminality. Children who have been abused (particularly physically abused) or neglected are more likely to end up as juvenile delinquents, likely as a result of a combination of the neurobiological and psychological effects of trauma and of a child's learning from the parent's example that violence is acceptable as a way of solving problems. This type of **social modeling** can also apply if children witness domestic violence, gang involvement, or other criminal behavior in the home. If parents are largely absent and do not supervise the child, this can leave the child to fend for herself and to be vulnerable to the negative influences of older peers or adults engaging in criminal behavior in their community. Parents who are present but use harsh punishment or rely predominantly on authoritarian or negative interactions with their child can also increase a child's risk for aggression and criminality. Finally, even with positive parenting and home life, exposure to community violence, gangs, and violence in schools can teach kids that they have to fight to stay alive, and make them feel criminal behavior is a necessary means to survival. Even if communities and schools are superficially safe, if a child feels alienated from adults and peers at school, feels he does not belong, and feels that adults treat him unfairly, he is more likely to become a bully or even to bring a gun to school.

Differential Diagnosis

As noted earlier in this chapter, psychiatric disorders are common in youths involved in the criminal justice system. Their symptoms range from mild to severe, with many stemming from family or environmental stressors or problems described earlier, such as abuse or lack of parental involvement.

Adjustment Disorder

Adolescents are vulnerable to stress when there are changes in their environment, such as parents' divorce (particularly if one parent is no longer involved with the child), a move to a new home or community, or the severe illness or sudden death of a family member. Adolescents can manifest this stress by acting out, particularly if they are impulsive and emotionally immature and thus unable to express their feelings verbally. Many adolescents will also cope with sudden stress by using drugs and alcohol, which can lead to arrest in itself or can increase their risk of engaging in dangerous or unlawful behaviors.

Attention-Deficit/Hyperactivity Disorder

The correlation between juvenile delinquency and ADHD is very high: approximately half of juvenile offenders carry a diagnosis of ADHD, and most of these youths have a comorbid diagnosis of conduct disorder (National Mental Health Association 2006; Teplin et al. 2002). ADHD can lead to delinquency in many ways. Children with ADHD are impulsive, hyperactive, and inattentive, leading them to act without thinking and often to be unaware or not conscious of the illegality of their actions and the consequences that may follow. Children and teens with ADHD also often get bored easily, have poor frustration tolerance and difficulty solving problems with peers or adults, and are more likely to use aggression or other impulsive acts to solve interpersonal problems. Teens with ADHD, particularly untreated ADHD, often experience academic difficulties (failing to complete their education; getting held back; having disciplinary problems, particularly if they have learning disabilities that are not being addressed in school) and are more likely to skip school or drop out (Stern 2001). If they are not in school, they are more likely to gravitate to gangs and other negative influences, and if they do not graduate, their job prospects are limited, leading some to get involved with selling drugs or other illegal sources of income. ADHD is also strongly genetic, and if a parent has untreated ADHD, he or she may have faced the same issues just described and may himself or herself be involved in criminal behaviors, such that there may also be a modeling or social learning component to the child's delinquency.

Oppositional Defiant Disorder

Some degree of argumentative and defiant behaviors toward adults is part of normal adolescent individuation. However, when these behaviors become persistent, pervasive, and keep the child from functioning appropriately at home or at school, a diagnosis of ODD should be considered. Individuals with ODD display an extreme and irrational presentation of argumentative and negative behavior. They are less likely to accept responsibility for their behavior, more likely to blame others for their problems, tend to perceive or attribute hostile intent to others (such as assuming an accidental slight is on purpose), and care less about the impact of their behavior on others. Many youths with ODD also have depression or ADHD, and about a third go on to develop conduct disorder.

Conduct Disorder

Children and adolescents with conduct disorder engage in deliberate acts of antisocial and/or potentially illegal activities; aggression; property destruction; theft; and violation of rules (e.g., truancy, running away, breaking rules at home or school). The younger the child starts engaging in the aforementioned activities, the worse the prognosis and the greater the risk of continued antisocial behaviors and violent aggression into adulthood.

Unfortunately, we do not fully understand what leads a child to develop conduct disorder. It is likely a combination of genetic vulnerability (including family history of antisocial behaviors as well as drug use, ADHD, or learning disabilities), exposure to physical abuse or neglect, parental psychopathology, poor attachment or placement in foster care, and broader community issues such as heavy exposure to gangs and community violence (Rosenhan and Seligman 1984).

Children and teens diagnosed with conduct disorder often exhibit academic problems (both learning problems and disciplinary infractions), lower IQ (particularly poor verbal abilities), difficulty understanding rules and empathizing with others, low frustration tolerance, and poor relationships with peers and adults (Huesmann et al. 1987). Adolescents are at an increased risk for suicide when conduct disorder, depression, substance abuse, antisocial behavior, ADHD, or trauma is present, and are even at further risk of suicide when arrested and incarcerated (Garland and Zigler 1993; Gould et al. 2003; Hayes 2004).

Alcohol and Drug Use

Teenagers often experiment with drugs and alcohol, but heavier use and earlier onset of use put kids at risk for negative outcomes, including delinquency. Boys growing up in poverty, those with abusive or mentally ill parents (including parents who use drugs themselves), and those with untreated ADHD, ODD, or conduct disorder are more likely to get heavily into drugs (Berk 2004; Teplin et al. 2002). Substance abuse and juvenile delinquency constitute one of the most correlated factors associated with juvenile criminal activity. When juvenile delinquents are arrested, they often test positive for at least one illegal substance, with marijuana, cocaine, and methamphetamines being the most prevalent, and nearly two-thirds of adolescents with legal problems have a combination of psychological and substance abuse problems (National Institute of Justice 2003; National Mental Health Association 2006).

Posttraumatic Stress Disorder

A majority of juvenile delinquents have a history of childhood abuse, witnessed violence (either community violence or domestic violence), and/or neglect, and many have PTSD and comorbid mental disorders (Abram et al. 2013; Cauffman et al. 1998; Steiner et al. 1997; Wasserman et al. 2002).

For some kids, their trauma and PTSD can predate and contribute to the delinquency. For example, if a child or adolescent was sexually abused, she may develop depression or anxiety, or try to numb her emotions through alcohol or illegal substances—and then end up arrested for drug possession. For other kids, the delinquency comes first and the trauma second—for example, when a youth with conduct disorder who is involved with a gang witnesses the shooting death of a close friend and then develops PTSD. Although the origin of the psychological problems within the context of PTSD may not always be clear-cut, the rates of comorbidity and PTSD are fairly high within samples of youths with juvenile delinquency. PTSD often goes untreated in juvenile delinquents and may contribute to additional victimization, further psychiatric issues, and recidivism.

Depression and Bipolar Disorder

Although many children may display symptoms of depression similar to those seen in adults (e.g., sad affect, anhedonia, self-esteem, concentration, sleep and appetite problems, suicidal ideation), many children and adolescents have a form of depression in which they are very irritable and can even be aggressive. Depression and other mood disorders (e.g., bipolar disorder) are common in juvenile delinquents. The high rate of these disorders may be related to the high rates of family and social problems faced by these kids, such as abuse, neglect, foster care placement, or lack of parental involvement.

Psychosis

Although psychotic disorders have been associated with criminal behaviors in adults, in children psychosis is extremely rare, and a child who is caught engaging in delinquent behavior and says "The voices told me to do it" may be trying to deflect responsibility. Psychotic disorders like schizophrenia generally start during late adolescence or early adulthood, and true psychosis in children and young adolescents is unlikely. The diagnosis of a psychotic disorder within the adult criminal population has been well studied, but there has not been a significant amount of research regarding psychosis within the juvenile delinquent population. Early signs of psychotic disorders in adolescents tend to look more like depression (social withdrawal, constricted affect, confused speech or thinking) and generally only later progress to involve hallucinations or delusions. Adolescents can, however, develop transient symptoms of psychosis (hallucinations, paranoia, disorganized thinking) if they are severely depressed, manic, or using drugs such as K2, "Molly," cannabis, cocaine, phencyclidine, amphetamines, or "bath salts." Adolescents who are high and experiencing hallucinations or paranoia are at high risk for violence. Many cases of drug-induced psychosis are short lived, and the individual returns to his baseline once the drugs are out of his system. Unfortunately, for some teens, psychotic symptoms can persist (particularly with marijuana and hallucinogenic drugs in kids with genetic risk for mental illness).

Identifying Immediate Triggers

Although these psychiatric syndromes, particularly if combined with other risk factors in the child and in the environment, can lead to chronically increased risk for criminal behavior, it is important to investigate whether the teen may have been "pushed over the edge" into delinquency by recent events at home, in the community, or at school. For example, a child with PTSD due to domestic violence at home might be a good student and generally doing well, and then brings a gun to school. Is he being bullied at school? Is he being harassed by gang members on his walk home? Has the abusive stepfather returned and the child took the stepfather's gun out of fear that, otherwise, the stepfather might shoot the child's mother? The interventions in this case will be very different than if it is a child who has always been a bully and who brings a gun to school to intimidate his peers and get his way. Even for a child like Adam, who has engaged in long-standing risky and delinquent behaviors, the immediate incident may have been triggered by drug intoxication or a recent fight at home. The child is likely to be guarded and resistant to talking about his motivations, but if you can take a curious and empathic stance (which is not the same as condoning the behavior), and also do some detective work to put the full story together, you can potentially discover why this dangerous behavior is happening now.

Risk Assessment

Any time a child is engaging in criminal behavior or gets picked up by the police, it is terrifying for those who care about the child. But by taking a moment to step back and evaluate the situation, you can assess the degree of risk and see how best to help.

First, has the child already been arrested or otherwise brought into the legal system? If not but you are concerned that she is engaging in criminal behaviors, you must assess safety and determine how to help the child while keeping those around her safe. If a child is engaging in heavy drug use, stealing, or truancy and it is related to problems or abuse at home, CPS should be engaged. If a child is engaging in these behaviors because of untreated mental illness such as bipolar disorder or psychosis, get him in immediately to see a mental health professional. If the child is already seeing a therapist or psychiatrist, do not assume that person is seeing what you see. If the child's behavior is endangering someone else, you may need to alert the parents, school, and/or law enforcement. By intervening quickly in these situations, you might be able to stabilize the situation and avert the child's getting arrested or worse.

If the child is already involved with the legal system, things can be more complicated. The legal system can be very convoluted to an outsider. Clarifying the charges, working with a lawyer to understand the child's rights (and yours), and determining the level and type of court involvement (including whether the child is being processed in the juvenile or adult court system) can lend some clarity. Most family court judges, police officers, probation officers, and even many criminal court judges are less interested in punishing kids (at least for minor crimes) and more focused on identifying the problems and getting the child on the right track. But the judge needs information and perspective on why the child might have gotten into criminal behavior and how those risk factors could be mitigated. If a teen has been resistant to mental health treatment or substance abuse treatment, a judge (with advocacy from the child's lawyer and information from mental health evaluations) can mandate the teen to intensive treatment that can prevent future criminal behaviors and perhaps save the kid's life. If a teen has been running the streets with a gang, stealing, prostituting, or engaging in other acutely dangerous behavior, and the teen's parent feels powerless to stop her, a judge might mandate the teen to a residential placement away from the negative friends and influences that first drew the teen to those negative behaviors. On the other hand, without information about how and why the child got involved in the criminal behavior, the judge might see the teen just as a "bad seed" and send her to a juvenile detention center that is unlikely to be therapeutic. Talk with the child, her parents, and their lawyer to see how to achieve the best outcome from this scary situation.

Finally, if the child is involved with the legal system and his parents are not the guardians or if the child is in foster care, it will become critical to clarify who has legal and decision making responsibility for the child. Knowing who the legal guardian is can also prevent mistakes and ensure you do not share private information with the wrong person. The child's lawyer (or, if the child is in child protective custody, the lawyer for the child protection agency or foster care agency) should be able to help you to clarify who has "rights" over the child.

Onsite Stabilization

When you become aware of at-risk, potentially dangerous, or criminal behavior with an adolescent or student you work with, there is much you can do to stabilize the situation in the community, to potentially avert the child's being placed in a jail or juvenile detention facility. There are a number of key factors to consider. Assess the risk factors and social and psychiatric issues behind the behavior; consider advocating for interventions such as diversion programs and individual and family mental health treatment; and develop an aftercare plan to manage ongoing risk.

Catch the Warning Signs

If you suspect or realize that an adolescent in your school, clinical, or pediatrics caseload is engaging in potentially criminal behavior, the first step is **assessment.** In school settings you see your students on a day-to-day basis, so you will notice whether there are changes in their demeanor or appearance, whether they are socializing with different peers, whether they have new academic and disciplinary problems, whether one of their parents was hospitalized or arrested, and so forth. If you are working in a pediatric clinic or therapy office, you will be the first to notice if there are unexplained bruises or broken bones; you will pay attention when parents or other colleagues also raise concerns about misconduct, possible drug activity, disruptive and violent behaviors, truancy, or mood changes in your patient or student. You may be able to understand the context for the child's behavior in a way no one else can. The child could be a victim, not just a criminal.

For Adam, there have been many warning signs—long-standing behavior problems, noncompliance with treatment, truancy, and substance use. Perhaps with the right services and help after one of Adam's earlier incidents of aggression or property destruction, the current crisis might have been averted. But many kids like Adam do not get effective help because the same risk factors that predispose them to delinquency make them challenging to help: they are distrusting of adults, in denial of their problems or need for help, confused about their current psychological and/or legal problems, manipulative, or straight-out lying to try to avoid their legal problem or some other family or social situation. They are likely to be initially resistant to your help, avoid eye contact, try to intimidate you or control the interview, or refuse to speak altogether. Many come from chaotic families or stressed, under-resourced schools where no one can take responsibility for them so they "fall through the cracks," with huge costs to the children and to the community.

Listen and Empathize

As stated above, adolescents who are engaging in criminal behavior or who are involved with the legal system are likely to be wary and resistant. While it is by no means easy, if you are patient and empathic and try to truly understand their history and perspective, without engaging in power struggles, these kids are more likely to open up.

Parents and guardians also need help, understanding, and empathy. Some parents will be shocked, as they had been unaware of the child's behavior, while others will be like Adam's parents, angry and resigned, saying they have been trying to get their child help for years to no avail. When you are meeting with the parents, try to get an understanding of the relationship and the dynamics within the family. Is the family involved? Have there been any recent changes in the family? Has the family been aware of the child's dangerous behaviors or concerned in any way? Is there a pre-existing issue? Are the problems getting worse? What steps have they taken to address the issue? Is the patient in treatment or taking medication? Does the parent dismiss or respond in a hostile or violent manner to the needs of the child? Is the parent psychologically and cognitively capable of understanding the child's needs? Is there a psychological and cognitive disconnect between the child's and the parent's behavior and temperament? Understanding the family functioning will be important in assessing the risk factors leading up to the delinquent behaviors and determining why the child and family have not gotten help before. It will also help to identify the strengths and needs of the family and child as they cope with this difficult situation.

Collaborate to Find Solutions

In trying to help kids involved in the legal system, remember that many parties may be involved with the child besides his parents and lawyer. In cases where the parents are not the guardians (if a judge has terminated parental rights due to abuse or failure to care for the child), determine whether the guardian is an adoptive parent, a foster care agency, or another child protection agency. The agency caseworker assigned to the child is likely to be able to provide this information. Even if the child's parents are still involved, the judge may assign a **forensic caseworker** to work with the family to monitor the family for the duration of the case and report his or her findings and observations (good or bad) to the judge. The child may also have a **law guardian** (a lawyer assigned to help represent a minor in court cases), a **guardian ad litem** (an individual assigned to a child in a court case when parents are not or cannot be present to represent the child's best needs), or a **probation officer** (who provides supervision of the child and gives documentation and information to the judge). Each of these individuals will have an important role and an important perspective in collaborating to find the best outcome.

Depending on where the child is in the legal system (engaging in dangerous behaviors or statutory offenses vs. facing actual criminal charges), **diversionary programs** may be an option. If the child is engaging in statutory offenses but not facing criminal charges, parents may ask the court for additional supervision through what is called a **PINS (person in need of supervision)** or **CHINS (child in need of supervision) petition.** A PINS petition is for a child under the age of 18 who has exhibited a reoccurring, pervasive pattern of disobedience (e.g., truancy, running away from home, extreme disregard for rules, dangerous behavior), and whose family has exhausted all possible measures of addressing the issue. The ultimate goal of filing a PINS petition is to provide the juvenile with diversion programs and move him away from at-risk illegal behavior, juvenile court, and detention.

If the child is facing criminal charges but they are not severe, diversion may be possible. The first step is for a **court program,** which is usually made up of child protection caseworkers and probation officers, to meet with the immediate family members concerned about the child and make appropriate treatment referrals. Certain therapeutic approaches have been proved to be effective for juvenile delinquents with mental health problems. For example, **multisystemic therapy** involves all the systems in a juvenile delinquent's life (e.g., family, school, community programs), and **functional family therapy** provides home-based treatment for at-risk juvenile delinquents. If the court program is able to provide the necessary tools for a juvenile to avoid court, then the child should be able to remain in the community. However, if juvenile has not utilized or cooperated with the court recommendations, or if any of the court orders are violated, the judge may decide to dismiss the request for a diversionary program and order the individual into treatment at a supervised facility or render a harsher disposition.

If an adolescent goes to court and is found guilty, he would be classified as an **adjudicated juvenile offender** and would be subject to carry out whatever disposition the court issues. A judge may decide not to incarcerate the juvenile but may order some combination of **restitution** (financial remuneration of damages), **community service, mental health treatment, probation or parole** (live at home but be monitored by the Department of Probation), **conditional discharge** (live at home without any further court supervision), or **verbal warning** about future ramifications if criminal behavior occurs again. Alternatively, the judge may issue an **adjournment in contemplation of dismissal (ACD),** in which the case will be dismissed after a 6-month period of acquiescence.

If the judge decides to **incarcerate** an adjudicated juvenile who was been found to have committed an illegal offense, the judge may order **house arrest,** may remand him to a short-term **juvenile detention center** or a **secure residential program** for an extended period, or may remand him to a **hospital for a psychiatric evaluation.**

Finally, for juvenile delinquents who have committed extremely heinous and violent crimes, a juvenile court may decide to relinquish their authority of the juvenile delinquent and transfer the individual to an **adult prison** to finish the remainder of the initial sentence or until he reaches the age of 18.

Learning From the Crisis

If a child or adolescent you are working with goes to court and faces one of the consequences discussed earlier, the problems are not going to disappear quickly; the child will likely return to your program, and your work will continue (unless the child has been transferred to an adult prison for an extended sentence). As someone who knew the child before the crisis, you can play a key role in rehabilitation, treatment, guidance, and supervision to try to avert further delinquent behaviors. The primary goal of your work should be ensuring everyone's safety and working to keep the child from escalating his behaviors and landing in the adult prison system. Unfortunately, when juvenile delinquents with mental health needs are sentenced to prison, these facilities are often ill equipped to meet the psychological needs of this forensic population. One of the many negative aspects of placing a juvenile offender in a prison with adult criminals is that he often emerges as being more criminally savvy and more violent and at increased risk of recidivism than juveniles serving time in juvenile detention centers. We all have an obligation to work with these teens and advocate for them to receive the right treatment so as to avoid such negative outcomes.

When to Get Help

If youths are engaging in risky or delinquent behavior that puts themselves or others at serious risk, or if they have expressed homicidal or suicidal ideation, emergency and police assistance is needed. Your first actions should be to de-escalate the situation onsite to keep the child, yourself, and others safe; notify other senior staff of the situation; contact 911; contact the child's parents; and accompany the child to a local ER for a psychiatric evaluation until the parents arrive. Your duty then becomes to communicate all the information you have, through a detailed letter or (ideally) a direct phone call, to the emergency staff who will be dealing with the case.

If you are concerned about an at-risk child but there is not an immediate risk, a referral to a clinician specializing in **forensic evaluation** is still often warranted. Although forensic evaluations are often court-ordered by a judge, forensic diagnostic assessment and consultation may also be requested by parents, the school, and treatment providers. Forensic evaluation is different from the consultation, evaluation, and treatment provided by a school psychologist, social worker, or therapist involved with the case. A formal forensic evaluation or consultation will involve integration of information from interviews with the child, family, and others involved, to provide objective, expert guidance on at-risk behavior, victimization, custody issues, diagnostic questions, or other issues important to the judge's decision. If you are involved in a treatment relationship with the child, you cannot also serve as a forensic evaluator, though the judge may ask you to testify in court as a **fact witness** presenting the facts of the case, the course of treatment, and any recommendations the court may need to assist with rendering a decision. Before responding to such a request, you should consult with your institution's legal team, because client confidentiality rules may require a subpoena before you are allowed to testify.

In the case of suspected child abuse, mandated reporters (e.g., a teacher, school psychologist, social worker, therapist, doctor) or a concerned parent may request that a forensic evaluation be conducted. When a child has disclosed abuse, or you have evidence to suspect abuse, the police and CPS are the first to respond and investigate an allegation of abuse. Child abuse cases are sometimes assessed by private forensic specialists, but oftentimes child abuse cases are referred to multidisciplinary specialized units, such as **Child Advocacy Centers.** These centers have specially trained clinicians who conduct child abuse forensic interviews and evaluations. These types of forensic evaluations are especially important when there is medical evidence but the child has not disclosed any information about the abuse.

For at-risk kids and adolescents, those engaging in status offenses, and those classified as juvenile offenders, the child's lawyer or the judge may require a **forensic risk assessment evaluation.** These evaluations review past violent behaviors and risk for future incidents. Risk assessment evaluations, which are typically conducted by mental health professionals, consist of review of medical, school, mental health, and legal records, followed by interviews with the patient interviews, collateral informants, and psychological testing. Furthermore, it is necessary to obtain a comprehensive understanding of the underlying psychological impetus, along with the pattern of criminal behavior, in order to assess the likelihood of the person committing a criminal act again and the level of dangerousness this individual might pose to themselves and others.

Managing Forensic Issues in the Emergency Room

If you are an ER provider and find yourself caring for a child or adolescent involved with the legal system, there can be many complicating factors to consider that are not at play with nonforensic cases.

Guardianship and Legal Documentation

If a child or adolescent is brought in by police, it is critical to ascertain who has guardianship over the child. Questions that may arise include

1. Who has physical custody of the child?
2. Do parents have joint or sole custody?
3. What if the patient was removed from the home because of abuse allegations?
4. If the parent has lost physical custody, does he or she retain visitation rights and/or medical decision-making authority for the child?
5. What if a parent is incarcerated and is unable to consent?
6. What if the child is a ward of a state?

The essential question is: Who has the legal right to make a decision about the child's psychiatric or medical care? This information will not only ensure the safety of the child but also reduce any potential legal ramifications between you and the family.

When parents do not have physical custody of their child but their rights and medical decision-making authority for the child have not been terminated, then clinical decisions and consent should be made directly with the parents. However, if a parent refuses to consent to a recommendation that is in the best interests of the child and that best ensures his or her safety, if parental rights were terminated, or the parent is unable to be present because of extenuating circumstances, then CPS would supersede as guardian and (after appropriate administrative procedures on their end) sign any legal paperwork pertaining to the medical and psychiatric issues until a permanent and legal solution can be arranged.

Forensic Cases in the ER

Children who present to the ER with police can be there for a **court-remanded psychiatric evaluation,** in **custody of the police,** or in **custody of either the adult or youth corrections system.** If the child is there on a court remand, the judge has demanded that the child receive a comprehensive psychiatric evaluation. Upon completion of the evaluation, the emergency doctor will determine if the patient may be held for treatment or discharged to the adult (usually either the parent or a law enforcement official) designated on the court remand. If the youth is there in police custody, it may be that he is being brought for a pre-arraignment hearing. Any juvenile delinquent with a past or current psychiatric history who is in police custody for a criminal offense must be psychiatrically evaluated prior to appearing before a judge for a pre-arraignment hearing. Unlike in other psychiatric emergency situations, an arrested juvenile delinquent will not be discharged to a guardian; rather, he will be discharged to the arresting police officer or member of law enforcement for arraignment in court, and if he needs inpatient treatment, that will likely occur in a specialized forensic unit. In many states this determination is made in collaboration with a specialized forensic professional. Finally, a youth may present to the ER for evaluation from a jail or juvenile detention center, in which case he is in custody of the **juvenile justice department** or the (adult) **department of corrections.** Understanding the legal status and custody status in such cases is critical for appropriate evaluation and disposition.

Unfortunately, many of the at-risk children and adolescents who enter into the juvenile justice system are provided with minimal opportunities for treatment or follow-up, which contributes further to recidivism risk factors. Our goal as professionals who deal with this challenging population is to understand the underlying cause or causes; reduce juvenile delinquency and recidivism rates through proper screening and interventions; challenge these youths' cognitive distortions; promote more effective coping and life skills; and help these youths shift their life course. Although this population can be challenging, research has repeatedly shown that with the proper professional support and treatment interventions, rehabilitation is possible for these children and adolescents.

References

Abram KM, Teplin LA, King DC, et al: PTSD, Trauma, and Comorbid Psychiatric Disorders in Detained Youth (NCJ239603).Washington, DC, U.S. Department of Justice, Office of Juvenile Justice and Delinquency Prevention, June 2013. Available at: http://www.ojjdp.gov/pubs/239603.pdf. Accessed September 14, 2013.

Berk L: Development Through the Lifespan. Boston, MA, Allyn & Bacon, 2004

Cauffman E, Feldman S, Waterman J, Steiner H: Posttraumatic stress disorder among female juvenile offenders. J Am Acad Child Adolesc Psychiatry 37(11):1209–1216, 1998

Cocozza J, Skowyra K: Youth with mental health disorders: issues and emerging responses. Office of Juvenile Justice and Delinquency Prevention Journal 7(1):3–13, 2000

Garland AF, Zigler E: Adolescent suicide prevention: current research and social policy implications. Am Psychol 48(2):169–182, 1993

Gould MS, Greenberg T, Velting DM, et al: Youth suicide risk and preventive interventions: a review of the past 10 years. J Am Acad Child Adolesc Psychiatry 42:386–405, 2003

Hayes LM: Juvenile Suicide in Confinement: A National Survey (NCJ 206354). Washington, DC, U.S. Department of Justice, Office of Juvenile Justice and Delinquency Prevention, 2004. Available at: https://www.ncjrs.gov/pdffiles1/ojjdp/grants/206354.pdf. Accessed September 14, 2013.

Huesmann LR, Eron LD, Yarmel PW: Intellectual functioning and aggression. J Person Soc Psychol 52:232–240, 1987

National Institute of Justice: Annual Report on Drug Use Among Adult and Juvenile Arrestees, Arrestees Drug Abuse Monitoring Program (ADAM). Washington, DC, National Institute of Justice, April 2003

National Mental Health Association: Prevalence of Mental Disorders Among Children in the Juvenile Justice System. Alexandria, VA, NMHA, 2006

Puzzanchera C: Juvenile Arrests. Washington, DC, U.S. Department of Justice, Office of Juvenile Justice and Delinquency Prevention, 2009. Available at: https://www.ncjrs.gov/pdffiles1/ojjdp/225344.pdf. Accessed September 14, 2013.

Robers S, Zhang J, Truman J, Snyder TD: Indicators of School Crime and Safety, 2011. Washington, DC, U.S. Department of Education, National Center for Education Statistics, U.S. Department of Justice, Office of Justice Programs, Bureau of Justice Statistics, 2012. Available at: http://nces.ed.gov/pubs2012/2012002rev.pdf. Accessed September 14, 2013.

Rosenhan DL, Seligman ME: Abnormal Psychology. New York, WW Norton, 1984, pp 720–735

Rutter M: Psychopathology and development: links between childhood and adult life, in Child and Adolescent Psychiatry: Modern Approaches. Edited by Rutter M, Hersov L. Oxford, UK,Oxford University Press, 1985

Shufelt J, Cocozza J: Youth with mental health disorders in the juvenile justice system: results from a multi-state prevalence study. Delmar, NY, National Center for Mental Health and Juvenile Justice, 2006

Skowyra K, Cocozza J: Blueprint for Change: A Comprehensive Model for the Identification and Treatment of Youth With Mental Health Needs in Contact With the Juvenile Justice System. Delmar, NY, National Center for Mental Health and Juvenile Justice, 2007. Available at: http://www.ncmhjj.com/wp-content/uploads/2013/12/Blueprint.pdf. Accessed September 14, 2013.

Steiner H, Garcia IG, Matthews Z: Posttraumatic stress disorder in incarcerated juvenile delinquents. J Am Acad Child Adolesc Psychiatry 36:357–365, 1997

Stern K: A treatment study of children with attention deficit hyperactivity disorder. OJJDP Fact Sheet 20. Washington, DC, U.S. Department of Justice, Office of Juvenile Justice and Delinquent Prevention, May 2001. Available at: www.ncjrs.gov/pdffiles1/ojjdp/fs200120.pdf. Accessed May 13, 2014.

Teplin LA, Abram KM, McClelland GM, et al: Psychiatric disorders in youth in juvenile detention. Arch Gen Psychiatry 59:1133–1143, 2002

Timeline of worldwide school and mass shootings, 2012. Available at: http://www.infoplease.com/ipa/A0777958.html. Accessed October 22, 2013.

Wasserman GA, McReynolds LS, Lucas CP, et al: The voice DISC-IV with incarcerated male youths: prevalence of disorder. J Am Acad Child Adolesc Psychiatry 41:314–321, 2002

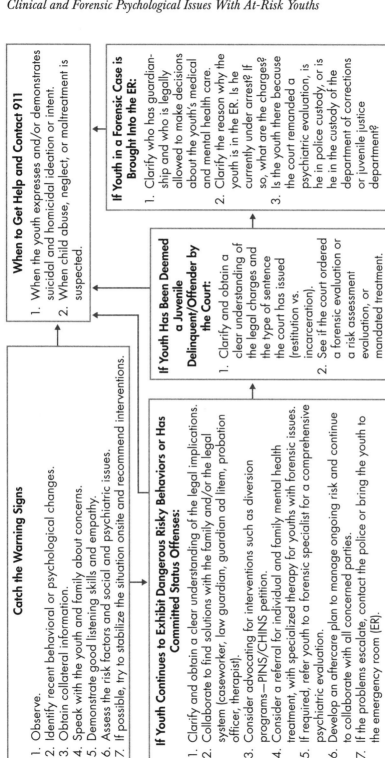

When to Get Help and Contact 911

1. When the youth expresses and/or demonstrates suicidal and homicidal ideation or intent.
2. When child abuse, neglect, or maltreatment is suspected.

If Youth in a Forensic Case is Brought Into the ER:

1. Clarify who has guardianship and who is legally allowed to make decisions about the youth's medical and mental health care.
2. Clarify the reason why the youth is in the ER. Is he currently under arrest? If so, what are the charges?
3. Is the youth there because the court remanded a psychiatric evaluation, is he in police custody, or is he in the custody of the department of corrections or juvenile justice department?

Catch the Warning Signs

1. Observe.
2. Identify recent behavioral or psychological changes.
3. Obtain collateral information.
4. Speak with the youth and family about concerns.
5. Demonstrate good listening skills and empathy.
6. Assess the risk factors and social and psychiatric issues.
7. If possible, try to stabilize the situation onsite and recommend interventions.

If Youth Has Been Deemed a Juvenile Delinquent/Offender by the Court:

1. Clarify and obtain a clear understanding of the legal charges and the type of sentence the court has issued (restitution vs. incarceration).
2. See if the court ordered a forensic evaluation or a risk assessment evaluation, or mandated treatment.

If Youth Continues to Exhibit Dangerous Risky Behaviors or Has Committed Status Offenses:

1. Clarify and obtain a clear understanding of the legal implications.
2. Collaborate to find solutions with the family and/or the legal system (caseworker, law guardian, guardian ad litem, probation officer, therapist).
3. Consider advocating for interventions such as diversion programs—PINS/CHINS petition.
4. Consider a referral for individual and family mental health treatment, with specialized therapy for youths with forensic issues.
5. If required, refer youth to a forensic specialist for a comprehensive psychiatric evaluation.
6. Develop an aftercare plan to manage ongoing risk and continue to collaborate with all concerned parties.
7. If the problems escalate, contact the police or bring the youth to the emergency room (ER).

Understanding clinical and forensic psychological issues with at-risk youths and juvenile delinquents.

CHAPTER 9

Substance Use

Helping Teenagers and Families Work Through a Substance Use Crisis

J. Rebecca Weis, M.D.
Stephen Ross, M.D.

Many people consider adolescence to be one of the least stable periods in the human lifespan. Add in the roller-coaster ride of drug and alcohol use and the instability suddenly multiplies. Unfortunately, drug and alcohol use is common in adolescence, and some youths even have their first drink or smoke while still in elementary school.

Drug and alcohol use in childhood and adolescence can interfere with the course of normal social and emotional development. During adolescence, the teen brain undergoes rapid development, with changes in wiring and connections between brain areas, and psychologically a teen is developing and consolidating his or her sense of self. All of this can be disrupted by substance use. We really know very little about the effects of illicit substances, tobacco, and alcohol on the teen brain during this period of extremely active neurological development. The research we do have suggests that there may be persistent cognitive impairments in those who started smoking marijuana as adolescents (Meier et al. 2012). And we absolutely know that adolescents are "experimenting" for themselves despite the lack of scientific data. The Monitoring the Future study and the National Survey on Drug Use and Health survey youths anonymously each year about their substance use, and the most recent data from 2012 indicate that 18.5% of 8th graders, 36.8% of 10th graders, and 49.1% of 12th graders have used any illicit drug in their lifetime (Johnston et al. 2013). Predictably, the percentages are even higher for lifetime alcohol use, at 29.5%, 54.0%, and 69.4%, respectively.

Case Presentation

Gina's parents walk in to your office on either side of Gina, who is 15 years old and looks sullen. Her parents ask to speak about something important. Gina's mother brings up that she thought Gina had smelled funny and her eyes had been bloodshot a couple of times in the past month when she came home on Saturday nights, but she and Gina's father really got concerned when Gina came home last night 6 hours after her curfew with her shirt ripped and looking like she would fall over any minute. They started trying to talk to her, but she blew up at them—she was so loud, they were worried the neighbors would call the police. She headed to the bathroom, saying she wanted to wash her face and go to bed. This morning, they found her lying on the bathroom floor, where she had slept all night. She could not remember if she had fallen or just lain down—thankfully she does not seem to have any injuries. Gina sits in the chair in the corner, glaring at her parents and avoiding eye contact with you.

Understanding the Crisis

When thinking about a case like Gina's, it is very helpful to think of adolescence as divided into three distinct stages, each with its own physiological, psychological, and interpersonal characteristics. It is important to understand these **developmental stages,** because how you talk with the child in front of you, and how you consider her risk for substance use, may vary considerably depending on the stage they are in.

Early adolescence—ages 11 to 13—is marked by the physical beginnings of puberty. Intellectually there is a growing capacity for abstract thought but a limited ability to think beyond the present moment into the future. Parents retain a very central position in the psychology of their children, but the drive to develop an identity of one's own leads to moodiness toward parents, demands for privacy, and susceptibility to peer influence. Because of this heightened sensitivity to peer influence and relative lag in ability to think into the future, young adolescents often make rather impulsive decisions based on what they face in the moment. Ongoing authoritative parental supervision is incredibly important when it comes to initiation of substance use as a counterbalance to peer influence. Early adolescents who spend a large amount of time without parental supervision and who are not involved in afterschool prosocial activities (such as sports or clubs) are particularly at risk. Initiation of substance use is particularly worrisome in this age group, since it is highly correlated with future addiction disorders (DeWit et al. 2000; Substance Abuse and Mental Health Services Administration 2012). For these reasons, if you have an opportunity to counsel young adolescents who have not yet experimented with substances, let them know how waiting even a couple of years can be seriously important to their future! And if you are aware of use already, there is certainly cause for concern. Alcohol and cigarettes are the most commonly used substances at this point, although marijuana use has been rising.

Gina is in **middle adolescence.** During this stage, between about 14 and 17 years of age, the adolescent continues to develop physically, ultimately achieving adult sexual development. Intellectual development progresses, with more ability to set goals for the future than previously–teens will begin to think more specifically about what they want to do after high school, and their goals become more realistic. Whereas a couple of years earlier in their lives many planned to be movie or rock stars, now they begin talking about becoming teachers, construction workers, lawyers, and other careers that are more attainable. They continue to develop their own identity separate from the identity they have formed within their family. They are often angered by the fact that they still have to rely on their parents and can be rather grandiose in their concept of what they can handle on their own. In addition to the continued importance of friends, they will develop special relationships with others of a romantic nature. They become increasingly interested in intimacy, and some (although not all) will become sexually active. During the transition from middle school to high school and then again from high school to college, one can see heightened risk for initiation of substance use as teens attempt to fit in with new peer groups and manage new stresses that overwhelm their current coping strategies. The same denial of risk that enables the adolescent to charge forward into the new challenges of each transition also can lead to risk-taking behavior with substances. By senior year of high school, 49.1% of students report that they have used any illicit drug, 45.2% report they have used marijuana, and 69.4% report they have used alcohol in their lifetime (Johnston et al. 2013). Because many teens are also learning to drive during this period, they need to be repeatedly informed about the dangers of driving while intoxicated–with alcohol, but also with marijuana or other drugs.

For most, adolescence does not really cease at age 18–and of course, when it comes to alcohol (at least in the United States), the legal drinking age is 21. By **late adolescence,** both males and females have achieved full physical maturity. Intellectually, most older adolescents have developed the capacity for abstract thoughts about topics such as philosophy, religion, and their own lives. The sudden and unpredictable shifts into immature behavior, common in early and middle adolescence, happen much less frequently. Proximity to parents is no longer so threatening, and a new adult-to-adult relationship emerges wherein parents and their offspring can enjoy one another as intellectual and emotional equals. Relationships with peers also tend to stabilize, and there is less need to "fit in." Older adolescents become more able to appreciate one another's individual characteristics, both positive and negative. During late adolescence, there may be less impulsive experimentation with substances, but binge drinking is prominent in college, so it is important to be aware to ask how much late adolescents drink at a time even if they drink infrequently. Blackouts can be an important indicator of binge drinking. For older adolescents who have already been using substances, this period of greater autonomy can also put them at risk for heavier and more frequent use.

Identifying Kids at Risk for Substance Use

Knowing about development will not suddenly make dealing with adolescents and substance use easy, but it is an important part of understanding the level of risk for substance use. There are also risk factors for substance use that are not dependent on the stage of development. First, there are several **environmental factors** to keep in mind. Youths from neighborhoods where substance use is prevalent are much more likely to start using. Part of this has to do with availability and access to substances (both legal and illegal), but these youths will also have more interactions with peers who are using substances.

Family history of substance abuse heightens the risk for not only substance use but also development of addiction through genetic as well as other influences. **Parental attitudes** about substance use also have an important impact on a teen's risk for using–although parents may not believe this, parental disapproval of substance use clearly factors in to adolescent decision making about substance use. **Lack of connection to other adult mentors** (e.g., coaches, teachers, religious leaders) is another risk factor for using substances. **Academic failure and poor engagement in school** distance youths from potential mentors and also contribute to a sense of hopelessness about attaining future goals, thereby increasing the chance that youths will choose a "good high" right now over success in the future.

Youths with **psychiatric symptoms and illnesses**, such as attention-deficit/hyperactivity disorder (ADHD), disruptive behavior disorders, depression, anxiety, and bipolar disorder, are also at increased risk to use substances. In addition, teenagers who have experienced **traumatic events** are at heightened risk for use and abuse of substances. This is true whether the trauma occurred in early childhood or more recently, particularly if it remains unresolved. Substance use may be the best way the teen has found to numb out overwhelming feelings and thoughts related to the trauma.

Differential Diagnosis

When approaching an adolescent who is suspected of substance use, there are two aspects of differential diagnosis to consider. The first is to clarify whether there is any other possible diagnosis (psychiatric or medical) that could explain the current presentation. The second is to determine whether there are any other diagnoses that make substance use riskier and more complicated for this particular person. It is also very important to recognize that there is a very high rate of comorbid psychiatric problems among adolescents who misuse and abuse substances, so assume there is something else going on until proven otherwise.

Adolescents occasionally come in asking for help on their own, having realized that they are using substances in a way that is getting them into trouble, but that is the exception rather than the norm. Adolescents who are using usually come to attention because family members, law enforcement, school officials, and occasionally friends have seen signs of intoxication and are concerned. Each substance has its own intoxication syndrome, so the following is certainly not a comprehensive list of possibilities, but rather covers some of the common issues that should be considered.

Medical Causes

In the case earlier in this chapter, Gina had either blacked out or passed out. But when an adolescent passes out, it is not always due to drugs: low blood sugar or cardiac arrhythmias might also be an explanation. Many of the symptoms of intoxication—confusion, slurred speech, difficulty concentrating—can also be symptoms of delirium, a medical syndrome with many potential causes (including substance abuse and withdrawal but also infections, very high or low blood sugar, and other medical illnesses). Thankfully most adolescents are physically healthy, but medical causes should always be considered, and if the adolescent has not had a physical exam in some time, it may be worthwhile to make sure one is done.

Kids who use drugs can also be at risk for potentially dangerous medical problems as a result of their substance abuse, such as dehydration, hyperthermia, seizures, or arrhythmias. MDMA (known as "ecstasy" and "Molly" among other names; see appendix to this chapter) can cause hyperthermia occasionally at dangerous levels; cocaine and amphetamines can cause seizures and/or cardiac arrhythmias, both of which deserve immediate medical evaluation. Some drugs can be life threatening during acute intoxication, including opioids (in particular heroin), alcohol, stimulants (e.g., cocaine, amphetamines, "bath salts"), and sedative-hypnotics (barbituates, benzodiazepines, γ-hydroxybutyrate [GHB], phencyclidine [PCP]). Particularly worrying from an overdose perspective are combinations of substances that can suppress breathing, such as alcohol plus opioids or benzodiazepines. Any of these situations or kinds of drug use warrant emergency medical attention.

Depressive Disorders and Bipolar Disorders

Both **depressive disorders** and **bipolar disorders** can lead to fluctuations in mood with accompanying physical symptoms that could at times mimic intoxication. There are important differences, though: the lethargy associated with "downers" (e.g., alcohol, opioids) and the hyperactivity and agitation associated with "uppers" (e.g., cocaine) will usually wear off in a few hours, whereas a central component of mood disorders is that the symptoms are persistent for a distinct amount of time. For example, major depressive disorder is usually only diagnosed if there have been a number of depression symptoms for at least 2 weeks. If an adolescent has been using substances *and* experiencing significant mood symptoms simultaneously, it may be worthwhile for the adolescent to have further evaluation with a mental health professional to assist in teasing these issues apart. It is also important to not assume that depression symptoms are only due to substances being used. Sometimes teens will attempt to self-medicate their depression with drugs or alcohol. This is particularly dangerous, because the risk for suicide is increased both in the context of depression and in the context of substance use in adolescents. Although low self-esteem is not a diagnosis, per se, it may be worth asking about it, because this can be a way that adolescents are able to talk about their depressive symptoms.

Psychosis

Many substances of abuse can cause hallucinations, paranoid thinking, or disorganized thinking or behavior that closely resembles psychosis. As with mood disorders, the time course and persistence of these symptoms can help differentiate those that are directly due to substance use from those that reflect deeper psychiatric illness. Keep in mind, however, that early in the course of **schizophrenia and other psychotic disorders,** it is not uncommon to see fluctuating levels of symptoms, and so the index of suspicion should be high in anyone presenting with psychotic symptoms that this might be more than a "bad trip." Marijuana, in the high-potency and synthetic versions currently easily available in most parts of the United States, has been associated with early onset of psychosis in those at genetic risk (youths with close relatives with psychotic illnesses). In one analysis, cannabis use increased the risk for clinically significant psychosis to one-and-a-half times that of cannabis nonusers, and the risk increased with more frequent use (Moore et al. 2007). A number of substances can also cause psychotic symptoms that persist for some time, even weeks, but these symptoms will eventually remit. PCP in particular has been known to cause such symptoms. Treatment of psychotic symptoms related to PCP with antipsychotic medication may be indicated in the short term, but the medication would ultimately be tapered off as the symptoms resolve. Co-occurrence of psychotic symptoms and substance use should be handled in consultation with a medical specialist familiar with serious psychiatric illness and substance use, given the complicated nature of these issues.

Attention-Deficit/Hyperactivity Disorder

Many substances can cause difficulty concentrating as well as physical agitation that can look a lot like the impulsivity and hyperactivity of ADHD. If you also learn from the history that some of these symptoms have been going on for a long time, consider the possibility that the adolescent may have ADHD. In fact, 23% of adults with substance abuse have ADHD (Van Emmerik–van Oortmerssen et al. 2012), and a childhood diagnosis of ADHD is known to increase the odds of developing a substance use disorder later in life (Charach et al. 2011). **Oppositional defiant disorder** and **conduct disorder** are also commonly co-occurring disorders and may themselves cause erratic behaviors that could be construed as substance intoxication at times. Importantly, all of these disorders have effective treatments and may respond to treatment better the earlier treatment is started, so early identification is very important. Despite initial concerns that treating ADHD with stimulants could increase risk for addiction spectrum disorders, a recent comprehensive review of the scientific literature, using meta-analytic techniques, found that treatment of ADHD with stimulant medication neither protects nor increases the risk of later substance use disorders (Humphreys et al. 2013). There is also some evidence that treatment of the ADHD reduces criminality and drug offenses, thereby perhaps at least reducing the drug-related harms (Lichtenstein et al. 2012). Treatment with stimulants is complicated once substance use has started (and sometimes even in adolescents who are not using substances but are at high risk to do so), however, because the stimulants themselves can be abused or sold on the street in return for other drugs. One approach is to use nonstimulant agents such as atomoxetine or to use long-acting stimulants to decrease abuse potential. Monitoring prescriptions and ensuring adult supervision of medication administration also play a role in managing the risk for abuse of stimulants.

Anxiety Disorders, Obsessive-Compulsive Disorder, and Posttraumatic Stress Disorder

While it is unlikely that most anxiety disorders would be mistaken as substance use disorders, many people with anxiety disorders, as well as obsessive-compulsive disorder and posttraumatic stress disorder (PTSD) (which, until recently, were included with the anxiety disorders in DSM), self-medicate with substances such as alcohol and marijuana. A recent longitudinal study confirmed that social anxiety was associated with later alcohol use disorders and that "PTSD predicted the onset of all substance use disorders" (Wolitzky-Taylor et al. 2012). Additionally, youths with severe PTSD may present with dissociative episodes and flashbacks that could be mistakenly attributed to substance use by those who do not investigate a little deeper. Obviously, asking adolescents about trauma exposure can be a sensitive topic, but in the context of suspected substance abuse adolescents really should be screened for past or current abuse (emotional, physical, and sexual). It is often best to reassure them before asking that you will not expect them to go into details right now but that you would simply like to know if there is any immediate danger in their environment so you can figure out with them how to improve the situation.

Substance Experimentation, Misuse, and Abuse

As was discussed earlier, degree of substance use occurs across a spectrum. According to the *Diagnostic and Statistical Manual of Mental Disorders,* Fifth Edition (also known as DSM-5; American Psychiatric Association 2013), a diagnosis of substance use disorder requires that at least two specific criteria be met. Examples of criteria include taking larger amounts of a substance than intended, a desire to cut down but an inability to do so, cravings, tolerance (leading to the individual's needing more than in the past to achieve the same effect), and withdrawal symptoms. The severity of the disorder can be classified as mild, moderate, or severe. Most would agree that experimentation with substances does not necessarily constitute a disorder—experimentation means that "use is infrequent and, in the case of teenagers, the substance is usually obtained from and used with friends in response to peer pressure" (Nelson and Stock 2014). Experimentation can become problematic, as in the case of binge use or use in dangerous or risky situations. It is also very important to be specific with the adolescent about the amounts being used—for instance, many of them have no idea that a half-full Solo cup of hard alcohol is actually at least four servings of alcohol.

Identifying Immediate Triggers

Assuming that you have determined with the adolescent that there is some substance use happening to cause the effects parents have been noticing, it is also possible that there is some acute stressor that is influencing the use. The substance use or other maladaptive behavior patterns are likely to continue unless the acute stressor is addressed. Sometimes, there may be enough symptoms related to the stress directly that the adolescent is suffering from an **adjustment disorder.** Common examples of these types of stressors include breakup of a romantic relationship, failing a test or class, bullying, and so forth. Even a simple problem-solving conversation with the adolescent can make a difference in such situations and may help you and the adolescent come up with some additional steps that could be taken by enrolling the support of others such as school officials or parents. In this case, substance use may be not only a way of coping triggered by the stress but also a cry for help in solving the problem. Also, if you get a history from an adolescent that he or she is using before school, be very suspicious that there is a problem with school—teenagers would not usually have reached such a degree of physiological dependence or craving that they would need an "eye opener" (as a morning drink is called by long-term alcoholics).

Risk Assessment

The most important first step in helping any child or adolescent in crisis is **acute risk assessment.** There are three main acute care considerations when dealing with a substance-using teen, all having to do with risks that could cause immediate and serious harm. Even one high-risk behavior or factor may influence your decision to have the adolescent assessed in an acute setting such as the emergency room (ER), whereas teens without these acute risk factors will benefit more from starting outpatient care with a therapist or drug-treatment program.

First of all, consider whether the adolescent is engaging in any **risky behavior while intoxicated.** Drunk driving is a serious cause of injury and death, but also ask about other activities that might be physically dangerous while the adolescent is intoxicated, such as riding bikes on the streets or getting into serious fights. Adolescents are also much more likely to engage in unprotected sexual activity when intoxicated and may be more susceptible to sexual assault. While asking them questions about their activity, you also have the opportunity to bring up the topic of birth control and protection from sexually transmitted diseases. Involvement in criminal activity is also certainly risky, but not always directly related to substance use. If the teen opens up to you about this, you should definitely factor it in to the risk assessment.

Second, screen for **specific high-risk substances or types of use** that have the potential for greater harm either immediately or in the long run. Ingestion of large amounts of alcohol in a short amount of time, which is relatively common in adolescence and definitely on college campuses, can cause alcohol poisoning. Alcohol poisoning can affect breathing, heart rate, body temperature, and the gag reflex. It can potentially lead to coma and death. If the adolescent has been experiencing blackouts, this may be a tip-off that he is engaging in binge-drinking episodes. Opioids also have the potential to suppress the nervous system to the degree that breathing is impaired. Heroin is especially dangerous, because batches of heroin are not standardized in potency. The same volume of drug that was safe the last time it was used could be fatal from another batch. The combination of alcohol and prescription opioids or benzodiazepines has also been involved in high-profile deaths of movie and TV stars—mentioning these young adults and their tragedies can help make this risk a little more real for the adolescent in front of you. You may not be able to convince a teen to stop using, but hopefully you can at least help him avoid really dangerous choices. Because prescription pills are not illegal, adolescents sometimes misperceive them as not harmful and may take quite large amounts in order to achieve a high.

Youths also use a number of ordinary household products, such as model airplane glue, cleaning fluids, and aerosol sprays, to get high through inhaling the fumes. Because the high achieved is very short lived, adolescents frequently inhale again soon after. Repeated use in a short interval can cause neurological toxicity, coma, and even death, especially with industrial solvents such as toluene. Some people may experience hallucinations and delusions as part of the acute intoxication with inhalants. This can also occur with PCP and crystal meth. Paranoia and agitation constitute a problematic combination, because violence and other erratic behaviors can emerge. The acute agitation and psychosis with PCP can persist for many days, leading to hospitalization for some.

Injection of any substance also clearly carries its own risks, including possible infection at the injection site (even with clean needles, since adolescents usually have not been instructed in sterile technique) or transmission of blood-borne pathogens such as hepatitis B and C and HIV (due to sharing needles). Aside from these physical risks, the method of administration can influence the risk for addiction—smoking crack and injection of various substances create greater risk for addiction because 1) the intensity of the high is greater, causing more craving for another high; and 2) the crash as the drug wears off is more unpleasant because it is also more rapid. Users are tempted to repeat their use to avoid the noxious experience of withdrawal. Certain substances also tend to have very high addictive potential regardless of the path of administration—crystal meth is a good example.

It is impossible to keep up with the risks of all the illicit substances available, because new drugs are constantly becoming available as dealers and users attempt to circumvent U.S. Drug Enforcement Administration regulations. Synthetic marijuana is a recent example. Adolescents are also creative in finding ways to get high and to get themselves in trouble. Recently, abuse of over-the-counter cough and cold medicines such as Coricidin and Robitussin DM has been popular among teenagers—taken in large amounts, the ingredient dextromethorphan acts as a dissociative hallucinogen, like ketamine. Such use can also be dangerous because cough-and-cold medications may also contain other ingredients, such as acetaminophen, that can be very dangerous in large amounts. In order to assess risk when an adolescent tells you he is using something with which you are not yet familiar, use the Internet. Please see the resource list at the end of this chapter for some helpful Web sites.

The third acute risk that should be assessed is **imminent danger to self or others.** Substance use is a serious risk factor for suicide among adolescents. Because of either underlying psychiatric diagnoses or the acute effects of substances, adolescents may experience urges to self-harm. Intentional or non-intentional overdoses usually require immediate medical attention; even if the adolescent states he feels fine, he may not be accurately reporting how long ago he took a substance, so you may not yet be seeing the full effect. This is especially true with pills, which of course take time to dissolve and be absorbed. The peak level of drug in the system may not occur for 1–2 hours or more after ingestion. Additionally, as noted earlier, some substances induce agitation and psychotic symptoms, leading to high risk for aggression. When this effect is very serious, the ER may be the only safe place to manage the adolescent until acute intoxication has resolved. Some drugs have antidotes that can be given to reverse the effects of the substance of abuse rapidly, but most do not—when antidotes are not available, supportive care, monitoring for medical complications, and administration of medications such as antipsychotics are sometimes necessary until the adolescent is sober again.

Although this chapter focuses mainly on acute management, Table 9–1 organizes some of the possible risk and protective factors that influence long-term risk for substance use.

TABLE 9–1. Risk and protective factors for substance use and substance use disorders

Domain	Risk factors	Protective factors
Individual factors	History of aggressive behavior from a young age Academic problems Undiagnosed mental health problems Child abuse or neglect Low harm avoidance and sensation seeking Antisocial behavior	Good self-control, coping skills, and problem-solving skills Mastery of communication and language skills Ability to make friends High self-esteem Engaged in positive pro-social activities
Family factors	Family history of substance abuse Lack of parental supervision and support Parent substance abuse Leaving home	Reliable support and discipline from caregivers Caregivers have clear expectations for behavior and values
School, peer, and community factors	Peer substance use Poverty Peer rejection Community norms favoring substance use Accessibility/availability of substances	Presence of mentors and connectedness to adults outside of family Opportunities for engagement within school and community Physical and psychological safety

Source. Adapted from National Institute on Drug Abuse 2003.

After you determine whether there are any acute risks, it is also important to consider how much risk exists for the substance use to continue and potentially escalate to a very serious problem. This will help you determine what level of treatment is likely to be needed by the teen. One of the biggest risk factors you will want to assess is **age at first use**–early use may mean that the teen already been using for years and is more resistant to stopping, and also increases the risk for eventual abuse and dependence. Additionally, if the adolescent is using one substance, he may be using others—you have to ask! As mentioned earlier, certain combinations could be acutely dangerous, but use of multiple different substances also probably means that the use is escalating in a way that may lead soon to a substance use disorder. Similarly, a rapidly escalating pattern of use, even of a single substance, is usually associated with development of tolerance, one of the symptoms indicating a substance use disorder.

It is equally important to look at protective factors, especially those you might be able to strengthen or promote. For instance, you can be the adult the adolescent connects to outside of the family and you can encourage the adolescent to stick with or join positive activities in the school or community (e.g., sports or dance teams, Boys and Girls Clubs, church groups).

Onsite Stabilization

If you have any hope of stabilizing the situation with Gina, you first have to try to find out what is really going on—but if you have ever had to deal with an angry adolescent, you know that the first thought that will cross your mind in this situation is "How in the world do I try to talk to Gina without her either lashing out or running away?" Although Gina is giving off many signals that she does not want to be here right now, she is here, which should reassure you a little. She has "allowed" her parents to drag her in. She is probably scared about what happened last night and likely has some conception that something worse could have happened—it is difficult for adolescents to admit being wrong to anyone else, but they can actually be pretty hard on themselves.

If you already know Gina and her parents, your next steps in handling this situation are perhaps a bit easier, but do not despair even if you have never met Gina or her parents before. You have already gotten a sense of what the parents are worried about. Although you probably want a lot more details from them, it is crucial that you start trying to talk to Gina soon. You are working against her natural and appropriate need to try to handle her problems without parents or other adults interfering. If she begins to perceive you as "siding" with her parents, she may feel less able to open up. After you listen to the parents' initial concerns, tell her parents that you are definitely interested in what they have to say but that you need to get Gina's side of the story before going any further. Ask them to wait in another area for a few minutes. If they protest because they are worried Gina will not be honest, thank them for letting you know about that worry and remind them that you will want to talk to them more, too. This is a nuanced discussion, but most parents will actually be quite respectful of you setting this boundary, as they realize deep down (under all that surface anxiety) that they need your help with this problem.

Once the parents are out of the room, you have to deal with confidentiality. You want to help Gina, and the only way she will let you is if she can actually trust you. It is complicated to deal with adolescents as they are transitioning out of the age when their parents know everything about them. Some parents have a very difficult time accepting this, so parents may need to be reassured that if there is anything going on that truly seems dangerous you will involve them. However, make sure they understand that there is too high a chance that you will get nowhere if you don't talk privately with Gina. You also have to let Gina know that there are limits to confidentiality in the case of actual danger. It helps a lot to tell adolescents that you will not reveal what they have told you without their permission except if you are really worried that they or someone else is about to get seriously hurt. Although adolescents tend to think of themselves as invincible, they also do actually understand that there are real dangers in the world, so they will usually accept these parameters without too much argument. It is also helpful to tell them that you will always try to let them know what is about to happen if confidentiality has to be broken and try to help them talk with their parents themselves instead of doing it for them.

If there is a high likelihood that substance use is the reason for the adolescent coming in, keep in mind that aside from confidentiality issues, the teen may be inhibited in talking with you because she assumes you are going to judge her harshly for using. Whatever your actual stance is about teens and substance use, you have got to find a way to contain your own views in the beginning and take a nonjudgmental stance. If you are struggling, it can help to remember that adolescents (and adults) often use substances to ease some sort of psychological distress—even though you do not condone the substance use, you are sympathetic to the pain that they feel. In order to communicate to the adolescent that you are not going to jump all over her when she tells you about what she is doing, you can just tell her! For example, you could try opening with, "Your parents seem pretty freaked out right now. I want to make sure you know that I'm kind of worried too, but I know that you don't need another lecture right now—you have permission to tell me if I accidentally start doing that." You are setting up a collaboration with the adolescent. If you are lucky, this may catch the adolescent off-guard, and she will suddenly be able to talk with you quite easily about what is really going on.

Sometimes, though, even your best lead-in cannot break through the resistance. Do not even try to break through forcefully—instead take a cue from motivational interviewing. **Motivational interviewing** is a style of counseling that was developed to help practitioners have productive conversations about change with individuals struggling with substance abuse (Miller and Rollnick 1991). Obviously you are not trying to help Gina change yet—you do not even know if she needs help changing or if she is actually abusing substances. However, some of the basic principles of motivational interviewing are extremely useful to open up the discussion: 1) roll with resistance, 2) express empathy, 3) support self-efficacy, and 4) develop discrepancy. If the adolescent does not answer your initial questions, roll into another topic or empathize that it might be really annoying having everyone make a big deal out of this. Asking teens about what music or movies they like can work as a topic—or look at what they are wearing and take cues about sports teams they might like. Then you can lead into whom they like to hang out with and whether their friends share similar taste in music/movies/sports. Circle around to asking whether any of their friends have been getting curious about alcohol, cigarettes, or weed. When the adolescent sees that you are calm hearing about other kids using, they really start to get it that you are not going to become overly dramatic about their use either.

Of course, in order to avoid getting dramatic, you need to be able to contain your own responses. Adults vary a lot in their opinions about substance use—and in their opinions about substance use in adolescents. Regardless of your own personal view, you probably care more about the health and well-being of the adolescent in front of you. You can maximize your potential to help her with whatever she is facing if you are able to maintain a nonjudgmental stance (or at least fake it well!). It helps to realize that your goal is to be neutral and sensitive in order to empower the adolescent to think about choices. You will not be with the teenager the next time someone offers her a drink or part of a joint, so how she thinks for herself is what really matters.

Catch the Warning Signs

Before we look at how to manage the adolescent who is already using substances in a problematic manner, let us consider whether we can prevent problematic substance use. On a population level, it is clear that **education** is key. For instance, cigarette smoking has decreased over the past several years in teens. This decline has coincided with an increase in teen's perception of harm related to cigarettes (Johnston et al. 2013). As teens are better educated about the risks of a substance, they are more likely to decide against using it. The United States has run a very successful campaign to educate the populace that cigarettes are associated with heart disease, lung cancer, and strokes. So if you are in an environment where you can provide information on substances to teens, either individually or in a classroom or group setting, it is worth doing so. It is important to avoid use of scare tactics, though, because that can alienate teens and discourage engagement. A balanced view of reasons people use and reasons people decide not to use is generally more effective.

On a more individual level, as noted earlier, adolescents all have a combination of risk and protective factors regardless of whether they have ever used. We can predict who will be at higher risk. If you are working with an adolescent who you recognize to be at high risk and have an ongoing relationship with that adolescent, let her know that you are willing to talk, if she ever wants to, about substances, peer pressure, or thoughts about using. If you can catch these warning signs, provide a supportive presence, and thereby help an adolescent decide to wait a little longer before trying something, you are helping her decrease her risk of addiction in the future.

If you know already that the adolescent is using, the first goal is to assess for any acute risk factors, including 1) current intoxication and 2) acute risk to self or others. You first need to know whether the adolescent is still intoxicated. Signs of intoxication of course vary by substance; some of the telltale signs for commonly used substances are summarized in Table 9–2. The Partnership for Drug-Free Kids Web site has a more comprehensive list (www.drugfree.org/drug-guide), including substances used less frequently by adolescents.

If the teen is intoxicated, the best thing you can do is make sure the situation does not get any worse. This means trying to limit environmental stimulation. Although you (or others nearby such as the parents) may have the urge to start lecturing right away on the dangers of intoxication, the teen may hear this as overly critical or aggressive. The teen might feel cornered and respond either aggressively or with self-injury. And at any rate, the teen is unlikely to absorb anything that is presented while she is in the intoxicated state, because the ability to process information is impaired. If the teen is responding preferentially to one person more than others who are present, that person can take the lead in the moment.

Listen and Empathize

Whether the adolescent is intoxicated or sober at the moment you are meeting her, she is unlikely to respond well if you start to lecture her about what she is doing *or* show a strong emotional response to her. The adolescent has probably heard it all before and has already had some adults get angry! Let the teen know right away that you are ready to listen and work with her to understand if there is any help she needs. You want to even the playing field with the adolescent to avoid getting caught in a power struggle. If she starts to let you know what she is using, be sure to understand what she likes about the substance. You may also find that she is using the substance to "treat" certain mental health symptoms, such as anxiety, or

TABLE 9–2. Some telltale signs of intoxication for commonly used substances

Substance	Signs of acute intoxication
Alcohol	Alcohol smell on breath, disinhibited behavior, talkativeness, dizziness, impaired coordination–at higher doses slurred speech, nausea, vomiting
Cocaine and amphetamines, including methamphetamine and "bath salts"	Dilated pupils, increased temperature, increased heart rate and blood pressure, insomnia, loss of appetite, restlessness and increased energy, irritability, anxiety
Dextromethorphan (ingredient in over the counter cough and cold medications, taken in large amounts to achieve a high)	Confusion, dizziness, double or blurred vision, slurred speech, impaired coordination, nausea and vomiting, rapid heartbeat, drowsiness, numbness of fingers and toes, disorientation, "plateaus" of hallucinatory experiences
Inhalants (effects are varied because most inhalants are actually mixtures of chemicals)	Slurred speech, lack of coordination, euphoria, dizziness–with repeated use, can see organ damage, including neurological damage; lingering headache could occur after heavy use
Marijuana	Problems with memory and problem solving, distorted perception (sights, sounds, time, touch), loss of coordination, increased heart rate, possible anxiety, bloodshot eyes, increased appetite, amotivation
MDMA (ecstasy)	Enhanced sense of self-confidence and energy, peacefulness, acceptance, and empathy along with involuntary teeth clenching, loss of inhibitions, focus on sights and sounds, nausea, blurred vision, chills and/or sweating; dehydration and hyperthermia possible
Synthetic marijuana	Lack of pain response, agitation, pale skin, seizures, vomiting, profuse sweating, uncontrolled body movements, increased blood pressure and heart rate with palpitations, possible dysphoria, paranoia, hallucinations
Opioids (including heroin and prescription opioids such as Oxycontin and Percocet)	Euphoria, flushing of skin, dry mouth, drowsiness, slow and slurred speech, slow gait, constricted pupils, droopy eyelids, vomiting, constipation

Note. MDMA=3,4-methylenedioxymethamphetamine.

to escape bad memories. Since substance use is frequently associated with mental health issues, it is important to ask about symptoms—most importantly, those that could lead to immediate problems such as suicidal thoughts or homicidal thoughts. If you are not accustomed to asking teens about mental health issues, doing so may seem a bit daunting at times; however, keep in mind that teens who are experiencing mental health issues have often been trying to deal with symptoms all on their own for a while. The stigma still surrounding mental health in our society causes teens to isolate themselves and suffer alone. Having a conversation about it with someone willing to talk for even a few minutes will be a great relief to most teens.

Collaborate to Find Solutions

You need to know whether the adolescent wants to get help. Although in certain situations you will determine that you have to force the issue and call her guardian or send the teen to the ER, there are many more times when doing so is not warranted and will only alienate her from seeking help—exactly the opposite of what you were hoping to do! As noted earlier, ask the teen what she likes about the substances she is using and then gently work the conversation around to whether there are any negative consequences for her. If she only sees the positives, try offering to show her some Web sites where she can learn more from reliable resources about the drugs she is using (some are listed at the end of this chapter). Remember the basic tenets of motivational interviewing—you have to try to develop discrepancy about the use of the substance while also supporting self-efficacy. This means that if you push too hard, you may get a commitment to change in the moment that will not be sustained even a little while later (because it came from you, not the adolescent). Believe it or not, even very brief interventions using motivational interviewing have been shown to have some positive effects, even as long as 12 months later, on problematic drinking behaviors (Bernstein et al. 2010; Monti et al. 1999; Spirito et al. 2004).

Learning From the Crisis

Depending on your setting, you may only have one shot to try to intervene. However, in many cases you will have other opportunities to work with the adolescent a bit later on. So maintaining the stance that you and the teen will collaborate to find the best solutions in the initial encounter helps you build the foundation for further growth. The concept of harm reduction can be helpful to consider here, since you usually will not be able to convince the teen in one sitting to become completely abstinent.

Harm reduction means focusing on reducing dangerous use (e.g., binge use, use in dangerous situations) when the "patient" is not ready to stop completely. You, as the helping adult, can at least help her avoid the types of use that can really hurt her while you continue to work on understanding the problem more in depth.

When to Get Help

If the adolescent is not acutely intoxicated and there are no acute psychiatric symptoms (suicidality, homicidality, acute agitation, or psychotic symptoms such as severe paranoia and hallucinations), you have a lot of options. If you have determined that the adolescent is experimenting without any serious danger for imminent harm, a little education from you may be all that is really needed. If at all possible, arrange for someone to be able to follow up in a few days to see how it is going. You may choose to maintain confidentiality (i.e., to not inform the teen's parents or guardians) to encourage follow-up and let the teen see that you trust he will continue to use appropriate judgment.

If the substance use is escalating or has reached a level that is beginning to indicate substance abuse *or* if you have uncovered comorbid mental health issues, some form of treatment is indicated. The teen's motivation to follow through plays a major role in how you choose to proceed. If the teen is really on board with the plan but does not want to involve parents (and you think this is safe enough), you may choose to refer to free self-help organizations such as Alcoholics Anonymous for teens. There are also versions of "Anonymous" groups for other substances, and information on these groups can be found online. If there are more worrisome risk factors though, or when there are comorbid mental health issues, a referral to formal treatment is likely indicated. If the teen is motivated to get help, you can likely collaborate with the teen to find a way to present this need to her parents/guardians without alienating the teen. Parents usually have to sign consent for treatment for teens, so this is an important factor in getting the teen into treatment. Also, parents are likely to see sessions popping up on health insurance statements, so they have to be involved on some level. Be prepared to talk with the outpatient clinician who is beginning to work with the teen to communicate your concerns and the plan you and the teen have developed so far. Also, if the teen is already in treatment, having begun prior to coming to you, consider getting consent from the teen and parents to talk with the current treatment providers. When those who are trying to help communicate with one another, the chance that the teen will actually be helped increases.

Sometimes there are serious concerns about substance abuse, but the teen just does not see it the same way you do. This brings you to a very difficult decision: whether to override the teen's desire to keep the use from parents/guardians or to respect that desire with the hope that the teen will at least come back to talk to you more about it. There's no one absolute answer to this dilemma. Keep in mind that the only leverage you really have is telling parents or sending the teen to the ER. If the teen goes to the ER while sober and is able to present well, there is a high likelihood that discharge from the ER will follow soon afterward. Sometimes the ER will provide some treatment referrals, and this can be helpful, in particular if you ask for help with referrals. This brings up the extremely important idea of communication with the ER. ER clinicians are very limited in the information they are able to collect most of the time; they rely on the self-report of the teen, who may begin to minimize substance use once he gets to the ER. If you communicate vital information to the ER clinician about why this particular teen is at higher risk, along with ideas about what may be helpful, the outcome of the ER evaluation will be a better service to the teen. Substance abuse treatment (as well as mental health treatment) is available on both outpatient and inpatient bases in most places. You may wish that the teen would receive treatment in an inpatient setting because you are worried that he will not address the problem any other way; however, keep in mind that this high level of care is reserved for those who have failed other levels of treatment (such as intensive outpatient rehab) and/or are in imminent risk of danger to self or others.

If in the process of talking with the adolescent you discover that there is an abusive situation in her life (which can certainly be the case) or she has encountered abuse while intoxicated, be sure to report this to the appropriate authorities. Especially in the case of sexual assault, evidence needs to be collected in a very specific time frame and ideally before the teenager has bathed or showered. To have this evaluation completed immediately is a good reason to send the teen to the ER immediately.

Other reasons to send the teen to the ER immediately, as have been previously noted, include acutely problematic intoxication, especially if there is concern for medical complications or serious agitation. Presence of suicidal or homicidal thoughts, as well as acute change in mental state or psychotic symptoms, should trigger emergency evaluation as well. Sometimes it may be possible for the parents to transport the teen to the ER, but most often in these very serious situations an ambulance is required.

Appendix: Some Common Drugs and Associated Street Names

Name of substance	Common street names
Dextromethorphan (ingredient in over-the-counter cough and cold medications, taken in large amounts to achieve a high)	Dex, Robo, Skittles, Triple C, Tussin
MDMA (3,4-methylenedioxymeth- amphetamine)	ecstasy, Molly, E, XTC, Adam, love drug
Marijuana	pot, grass, weed, reefer, skunk, ganja
Synthetic marijuana	Spice, K2, fake weed, skunk, moon rocks
Prescription opioids	Oxy, OC, percs, vikes, happy pills
PCP (phencyclidine)	Angel dust, killer weed, wack, ozone

References

American Psychiatric Association: Diagnostic and Statistical Manual of Mental Disorders, 5th Edition. Arlington, VA, American Psychiatric Association, 2013

Bernstein J, Heeren T, Edward E, et al: A brief motivational interview in a pediatric emergency department, plus 10-day telephone follow-up, increases attempts to quit drinking among youth and young adults who screen positive for problematic drinking. Acad Emerg Med 17:890–902, 2010

Charach A, Yeung E, Climans T, Lillie E: Childhood attention-deficit/hyperactivity disorder and future substance use disorders: comparative meta-analyses. J Am Acad Child Adolesc Psychiatry 50:9–21, 2011

DeWit DJ, Adlaf EM, Offord DR, Ogborne AC: Age at first alcohol use: a risk factor for the development of alcohol disorders. Am J Psychiatry 157:745–750, 2000

Humphreys K, Eng T, Lee S: Stimulant medication and substance use outcomes: a meta-analysis. JAMA Psychiatry 70:740–749, 2013

Lichtenstein P, Halldner L, Zetterqvist J, et al: Medication for attention deficit-hyperactivity disorder and criminality. New Engl J Med 367(21):2006–2014, 2012

Johnston LD, O'Malley PM, Bachman JG, Schulenberg JE: Monitoring the Future National Survey Results on Drug Use, 1975–2012: 2012 Overview–Key Findings on Adolescent Drug Use. Available at: http://www.monitoringthefuture.org/pubs/monographs/mtf-overview2012.pdf. Accessed January 21, 2014.

Meier M, Caspi A, Ambler A, et al: Persistent cannabis users show neuropsychological decline from childhood to midlife. Proc Natl Acad Sci USA 109:E2657–E2664, 2012

Miller WR, Rollnick S: Motivational Interviewing: Preparing People to Change Addictive Behavior. New York, Guilford, 1991

Monti PM, Colby SM, Barnett NP, et al: Brief intervention for harm reduction with alcohol-positive older adolescents in a hospital emergency department. J Consult Clin Psychol 67:989–994, 1999

Moore TH, Zammit S, Lingford-Hughes A, et al: Cannabis use and risk of psychotic or affective mental health outcomes: a systematic review. Lancet 370:319–328, 2007

National Institute on Drug Abuse: Preventing drug use among children and adolescents (In Brief), Revised (NIH Publ No 04-4212[A]), October 2003. Available at: http://www.drugabuse.gov/publications/preventing-drug-use-among-children-adolescents. Accessed January 21, 2014.

Nelson GA, Stock C: Stages of substance abuse, in Health Encyclopedia. Rochester, NY, University of Rochester Medical Center. Available at: http://www.urmc.rochester.edu/encyclopedia/content.aspx?ContentTypeID=1&ContentID=3060. Accessed July 15, 2014.

Spirito A, Monti PM, Barnett NP, et al: A randomized clinical trial of a brief motivational intervention for alcohol-positive adolescents treated in an emergency department. J Pediatr 145(3):396–402, 2004

Substance Abuse and Mental Health Services Administration: Results from the 2010 National Survey on Drug Use and Health (NSDUH), January 2012. Available at: http://www.samhsa.gov/data/NSDUH/2k10MH_Findings/2k10MHResults.htm. Accessed January 21, 2014.

Van Emmerik–van Oortmerssen K, van de Glind G, van den Brink W, et al: Prevalence of attention-deficit hyperactivity disorder in substance use disorder patients: a meta-analysis and meta-regression analysis. Drug Alcohol Depend 122:11–19, 2012

Wolitzky-Taylor K, Castriotta N, Lenze EJ, et al: Longitudinal investigation of the impact of anxiety and mood disorders in adolescence on subsequent substance use disorder onset and vice versa. Addict Behav 37:982–985, 2012

Online Resources

Partnership for Drug-Free Kids
> http://www.drugfree.org/drug-guide (Good resource to look up drugs with which you may not yet be familiar)
> http://www.drugfree.org and http://timetoact.drugfree.org/think-first-step-ask.html

Alcoholics Anonymous for teenagers
> http://www.aa.org/lang/en/catalog.cfm?origpage=15andproduct=94

National Institute on Drug Abuse (NIDA) (for teens)
> http://www.teens.drugabuse.gov

National Institute on Alcohol Abuse and Alcoholism (NIAAA)
> http://www.niaaa.nih.gov

Substance Abuse and Mental Health Services Administration (SAMHSA)
> http://www.samhsa.gov

Center for Adolescent Substance Abuse Research (CeASAR)
> http://www.ceasar-boston.org and www.Teen-Safe.org

Catch the Warning Signs

1. If the teen is at high risk for substance abuse, try to preemptively counsel.
2. Encourage prosocial activities and other protective factors (see Table 9–1).
3. Assess for other mental health issues and refer for treatment.
4. If the teen shows signs of intoxication, provide a calm environment while evaluating for other acute risks.

De-escalation: Listen and Empathize

1. Avoid lectures or angry responses.
2. Ask the teen what she likes about the substance.
3. Assess again for comorbid mental health issues.

If the Teen Shows Evidence of Any Toxicity or Acute Psychiatric Risk:

1. Call for help.
2. Physically contain the teen if you must to maintain safety.

Refer to the Emergency Room if:

1. Agitation is unmanageable.
2. There is risk of acute toxicity from substance used.
3. The teen expresses suicidal/homicidal ideation, threats.
4. There are serious psychotic symptoms.
5. There is recent or ongoing abuse, including sexual assault.

De-escalation: Collaborate for Solutions

1. Ask the teen if the substance has any negatives.
2. Assess whether the teen would like help.
3. Support self-efficacy while you help develop discrepancy.

De-escalation

Learn from the crisis
1. Consider harm reduction strategies.
2. Plan to talk again soon.

Make referrals if:
1. Substance use is escalating.
2. There are serious risks with substances used:
   a. Risky behaviors while intoxicated.
   b. Risk of serious harm from the substance.
   c. Risk of serious harm from mode of administration.
3. There are comorbid mental health issues.

Managing substance abuse risk and crisis.

CHAPTER 10

Finding Help

Helping Families Find Effective Treatment for Children With Psychiatric Illness

Jasmine Marrero, LCSW

Melissa Negron, LCSW

Maggie Bielsky, LMSW

In any given year, only 20% of children with psychiatric illness receive the treatment they need (U.S. Public Health Service 2000). Unfortunately, there are many barriers to children receiving the right care, including barriers to accessing treatment (due to issues related to insurance, financial resources, or availability of trained providers in the area), lack of understanding of mental illness and the need for treatment on the part of the family or child, and difficulties navigating our complex mental health system, particularly for children whose families are poor and children in the foster care system. By understanding the different overlapping service systems in which children's mental health treatment can be provided, you can be a more effective advocate for children to get the care they need and deserve.

We would like to thank Maria Gandolfo for her contribution to our chapter.

Case Presentation

Kassandra, age 9, presents to the emergency room (ER) for a psychiatric evaluation, accompanied by her mother. Since her father was deported to Ecuador 3 months ago, Kassandra, her mother, and her two younger siblings have been forced to relocate to a community shelter and transfer to a new school. Kassandra's mother is currently unemployed, and she has no family or friends nearby. At home, Kassandra's mood swings wildly between sadness and irritability, with bouts of crying, shouting, and slamming doors when upset. Since arriving at the shelter, she has lost five pounds and does not sleep well because of nightmares. At school, teachers have reported that she is often inattentive, anxious, impulsive, and easily frustrated, particularly in classes that may be more challenging for her such as reading and math. She is prone to have meltdowns if there is a change in her routine or a sudden transition; in these moments she runs out of class, often to be found sitting in the corner of an empty classroom, unresponsive, biting herself and rocking back and forth. Her behavior at school has placed her in jeopardy of being held back, while the shelter staff are threatening to remove the family from the shelter or recommend that Kassandra be placed in foster care.

Kassandra's mother, who has struggled with depression in the past, is feeling overwhelmed by Kassandra's needs, those of her two younger children, and the broader stressors of financial strain, lack of permanent housing, lack of child care, and lack of a support system. Kassandra's mother feels isolated and alone and worries how this may impact her ability to effectively parent her children and meet even their basic needs.

Understanding the Crisis

Kassandra's story demonstrates the complicated interactions among psychosocial stressors, mental illness, and the difficulties of navigating complex systems to find appropriate treatment in the community. When thinking about cases like Kassandra's, it is useful to consider the four areas of the social services systems that affect children: mental health, education, child welfare, and developmental disabilities.

Because the nature and availability of these services vary from state to state, we advise our readers to familiarize themselves with the resources specific to their location. We will generally focus on services offered in New York State, but most localities will have programs analogous to the services discussed in each section. Services identified, or those analogous to the ones discussed, can be accessed by contacting the program directly or through your local hospital, state or local government mental health agency, designated hotline, or department of children and families.

Mental Health Services

Most people, when they think of mental health treatment, think of inpatient units or outpatient mental health clinics, but actually the mental health system consists of a broad set of interconnecting services. **Outpatient mental health clinics** generally offer a broad range of programs for individual, family, and group therapy to address a range of psychiatric problems. Unfortunately many clinics have wait lists and lengthy intake processes, so some outpatient clinics offer **walk-in services** or **crisis clinics** to allow faster access to treatment for situations that are urgent but not emergencies. Sometimes these clinics are connected to ERs, and children can be seen there after having been to an ER in crisis, while in other hospital systems these clinics are freestanding or based in an outpatient treatment center. These clinics generally focus on rapid assessment of the child's and family's needs, providing psychoeducation, improving coping skills, establishing a support network, improving self-care, and engaging in a discussion of continued psychiatric care.

School-based clinics provide support to students in an easy-to-access, school-based setting. Schools are often where mental illness and other disabilities are first recognized and addressed; of the 16% of children in the United States who receive mental health services, 70%–80% of them receive these services at school. School-based clinics generally offer individual, group, and family therapy, and some even have an on-staff psychiatrist or registered nurse to provide, prescribe, and manage psychiatric medications. School-based clinics often also collaborate with school psychologists to care for children with learning disabilities, behavioral or emotional problems, or developmental disorders, such as autism. In some communities the school-based clinic is physically located in the school, while in other communities there is a mobile team that may cover several schools. Often there is 24-hour telephone coverage to address crises that occur outside of the school day, and the clinics are often accessible during the summer and holidays. To see if such a program is available in your area, contact your local school district.

Sometimes, in complicated cases like Kassandra's, a family needs more help than can be given in once- or twice-a-week office visits. A number of additional mental health resources may be available, and depending on the needs of the individual child and family, one or more programs might be the best fit.

Community Supports for Families

Navigating and accessing services in the community can be very overwhelming and intricate. Many states support **community resources** that provide advocacy for parents, including assistance in care coordination with child welfare services; family court; school meetings; medical/therapy appointments; linkage to other supportive services; clinical consultation and supportive counseling to families; workshops; and educational and parenting services; as well as respite programs. Often programs are staffed with **family advocates** who have experience with getting services for their own children and can work with the family more holistically and provide parents with necessary tools and support. The advocates are available to accompany and assist parents in navigating systems such as board of education, child welfare, juvenile justice, and mental health while ensuring that parents are aware of their rights (NYC Department of Education 2013). If your community does not have a stand-alone program like this, NAMI (National Alliance on Mental Illness) provides online trainings, support, and advocacy resources.

Crisis Services

Even with outpatient treatment and community supports, families may still need help in a crisis. While ERs are always available, there can be long waits, children may be frightened by the chaos and white coats, and ER staff may not be trained in helping children and families specifically with psychiatric problems. To address this, the mental health system generally offers a number of other crisis services that may be useful. These differ from state to state but generally fall into a few models of care.

Mobile crisis programs provide rapid psychiatric assessment and treatment outside of the ER setting (NYC Department of Health and Mental Hygiene 2012c). Mobile teams can be made up of different staff but often have a team of mental health professionals (which may include a psychiatrist, psychologist, nurse, social worker, and/or caseworker) who work together to assess and stabilize the patient. In some states (e.g., Massachusetts) the mobile crisis team responds immediately to a crisis call, while in others (e.g., New York) they provide more subacute care, seeing the patient within 24–48 hours of the call and then following him or her over the course of three to six visits. Mobile crisis teams meet the patient in the community, often in his or her home or school (though some programs will go to an emergency room to evaluate a patient there), and can also meet with family members or others involved with the patient. They assess the patient, both for safety and more generally for psychiatric diagnosis and need for treatment, and then help the patient and family to access the right types of treatment and services.

Home-based crisis programs provide in-home, intensive treatment, generally for a limited period of time (usually weeks to months), for families with a child who is experiencing severe difficulties and is at risk for hospitalization (NYC Department of Health and Mental Hygiene 2013). Some are provided through foster care agencies, while others are open to kids still living with their families of origin. Treatment takes place in the home, at school, or in the community and usually involves multiple visits per week with the therapist, the child, and the family. Often the therapist is also available by phone for help in a crisis. The therapist will assess the child's and family's needs; provide treatment, including developing coping skills and strategies in managing conflicts both in the home and in the community; work to improve the family's communication with and support of the child; and help the family connect to other community-based resources and supports and collaborate with those other resources if they are already in place.

Case Management

Unfortunately, children with severe mental illness can be at risk for repeated crises and multiple hospitalizations. Many states or insurance programs provide **case management** services to give guidance and oversight in high-risk or complex cases over an extended period of time. For a case like Kassandra's, in which the mother is overwhelmed and does not understand all the services available to her, case management can be really useful. In many states, different levels of case management services are available, ranging from more intense to less intense depending on the needs of the child and family. The less intense programs, often called **supportive case management,** may involve monthly or twice-monthly meetings with a case manager to ensure the child is staying connected to treatment. Higher-risk cases will be assigned an **intensive case manager,** who is available 24 hours a day, 7 days a week, and who will see the family at least four times per month. Sometimes case managers work as a team, providing more flexible levels of support for children whose needs fluctuate (NYC Department of Youth and Community Development 2011).

One very important, national case management program is the **Home and Community-Based Services** (HCBS) Waiver program, available to states under the Medicaid Program. The HCBS Waiver program serves children with serious emotional disturbances that interfere with their daily functioning. This intensive program combines case management, home-based therapies, individualized care coordination, respite care, skill-building services, family support, and intensive in-home and crisis response for children and adolescents ages 5–17. Although many referrals to these programs are generated from psychiatric inpatient settings, patients can also be referred to these types of services by community therapists, schools, child welfare workers, and juvenile justice systems. Many states have a centralized referral process (in New York State it is called the Children's Single Point of Access, or CSPOA) to streamline the process of getting connected (NYC Department of Health and Mental Hygiene 2012a). These services can often provide the supports and treatment that a child needs to avoid ER visits and hospitalizations that disrupt his home and school lives.

Out-of-Home Mental Health Treatment

Unfortunately, some children need long-term, very intensive mental health treatment, beyond a short-term hospitalization but also beyond what a family can provide at home. For these children, a residential program may be a necessary step for stabilization before they are able to go home. Sometimes these services are accessed on discharge from the hospital, and sometimes a child is put into one of these programs to stabilize her so she does not worsen and need hospitalization.

Children's community residences are small therapeutic residential programs within the community that house up to eight children and youths between ages 5 and 18 years who present with serious emotional and behavioral dysregulation and are unable to remain at home (NYS Department of Health and Mental Hygiene 2012b). Preferably, participants are placed in residences close to their homes so as to provide accessibility for family and caregivers. Emphasis is placed on the importance of working with family members and the participant in developing skills, establishing supports and improving relationships that will result in the child/youth returning to her home or preparing for independent living. Programs offer a therapeutic milieu that includes structured daily living activities, problem solving skills training, and behavioral management. Participants can attend their neighborhood schools and take part in local recreational and cultural programs, all under the close supervision of specially trained staff. Lengths of stay vary based on the participants' needs.

Residential treatment facilities are residential psychiatric facilities that provide comprehensive mental health and educational services for children and youths. Many have age cutoffs (usually ages 5–21) and also generally require participants to have an IQ over 50 (NYC Department of Health and Mental Hygiene 2012b). The participants must present with a serious emotional disturbance and have demonstrated that they cannot be safely maintained within the home or community, thus requiring a comprehensive longer-term inpatient treatment program. Services include case coordination, crisis intervention, medication management, various forms of therapy (e.g., individual, group, art), recreation, skill building, and educational/vocational training. Referrals to these facilities are made only after other appropriate community-based programs have been attempted, considered, and/or ruled out, because it is always better for a child to remain with his or her family whenever possible.

The Department of Education

Risk Assessment

When we are confronted with a case like Kassandra's, it is important to consider whether any academic difficulties or learning disabilities are contributing to her difficult behaviors. Kassandra has had persistent difficulties in reading and math, as well as symptoms consistent with attention-deficit/hyperactivity disorder and a possible learning disorder—all of which have gone undetected and undiagnosed. Outpatient psychiatric treatment can address some of these issues, but she will also need additional services and supports through the educational system.

School-Based Interventions

There are several types of school-based services that Kassandra may be eligible for, and as a clinician working with children who have psychiatric diagnoses, you will find it helpful to become familiar with these services and how you can advocate in obtaining the appropriate school-based interventions. The first step is an educational assessment to understand the child's strengths and weaknesses in areas of intelligence, attention, problem solving, memory, personality, motor, language, and perceptual and learning abilities. Testing can also provide guidance in which interventions would be helpful.

Individualized education plan.   Children like Kassandra need special academic supports and modifications, which should be laid out in an **Individualized Education Program, or IEP.** The first step to obtaining an IEP is to identify the child as requiring a special education and/or related services. A child can be identified by a teacher or school professional, a parent, or even an outside professional such as a doctor, therapist, social worker, or case manager, but it is the parent who must formally request an IEP. As a clinician working with a child or family outside of the school system, you will find it prudent to counsel parents in obtaining an IEP when a child's disability appears to be affecting his ability to function behaviorally or academically in the school setting (Price-Ellingstad et al. 2000).

The request should be made in writing and given to the IEP coordinator at the school. The child will then undergo an educational assessment by a professional appointed by the school district. This assessment may also include evaluations completed by the child's psychiatrist, therapist, or pediatrician. Observations made by parents, teachers, and other school staff are also a vital part of the educational evaluation. Once the child is evaluated and determined eligible, the IEP team must develop the IEP within 30 calendar days of the child's being deemed eligible (Price-Ellingstad et al. 2000).

The IEP outlines school-based services, supports, and special education plans for children with different types of disabilities. In this case a disability can be an emotional disability, a learning disability, a developmental disability, or another medical condition (such as seizures or blindness) that may prevent the student from accessing education. The document also outlines how these interventions will be implemented and how progress and outcomes will be measured and tracked. The IEP is created in collaboration with parents; in some cases, the identified student; teachers; and other related school staff, such as school social workers, guidance counselors, school psychologists, and principals. At times, outside treatment providers such as pediatricians, therapists, and other clinicians may be asked or may want to participate in the development of their patient's/client's IEP. These individuals will come together to provide input regarding concerns and solutions in order to develop the IEP. Once the IEP is in place, the child's progress is regularly measured, and reports should be provided to families and the students must be reevaluated once every 3 years, but the students can be reevaluated more often as requested by parents or school staff (Price-Ellingstad et al. 2000).

If parents are having difficulty getting the right IEP services for their child, it may also be helpful to connect the child's family with a parent advocate or parent coordinator. These professionals assist parents in navigating the services that are provided by the public school system, connect them to helpful resources, and help to address any concerns the family may have. A request for a parent advocate or coordinator can be made either through the school's administrative office or through the district office. Most public school districts provide this service for families (NYC Department of Education 2013).

Special education services can be provided in a range of settings, depending on the needs of the child:

> **General education setting:** Children who receive special education services in a general education setting take classes with the general population of their school while receiving supplementary aids and services called **accommodations.** Examples of accommodations are being able to take notes on a computer, use a calculator in math, have large-print or Braille materials, listen to a book on tape as opposed to having read a book, or other specific changes. Students may also receive **modifications in the curriculum,** which are actual alterations of the instruc-

tional level with content remaining the same (Massachusetts General Hospital 2010). An example of a modification would be reducing the length of a book report for a student with a reading disorder. Students may benefit from other supports, such as being granted extended time to take tests, sitting in the front of the class or near the teacher, being allowed to get up and move around at certain times, being offered repetition or rephrasing of instructions, and having access to organizational aids, additional notes, and study guides. Some students may receive **related services** outside of the classroom setting, such as counseling, speech therapy, occupational therapy, audiological services, health services, physical therapy, vision services, mobility services, or the services of an individual paraprofessional, who can assist a student in behavior management, health, transportation, self-care, or interpretation services. Students can also be pulled out of the general classroom setting to be provided with additional instruction by a special education teacher, which can be administered individually or in a group setting. Or the special education teacher can provide consultation in how instruction can be delivered (Price-Ellingstad et al. 2000). Kassandra would most likely benefit the most from this general education setting, which would allow her to stay in her own classroom in order to prevent yet another stressful transition. However, if Kassandra cannot get enough services in this setting, her IEP might be revised to move her to either an Integrative Co-Teaching classroom or a self-contained or special education classroom.

Integrated Co-Teaching classroom (also known as *collaborative team teaching*): In this setting, students with and without disabilities are team-taught by a general education teacher and a special education teacher. Both teachers collaborate to provide modified curriculum so that each student has access to the general education curriculum (NYC Department of Education 2009).

Self-contained or special education classes: This setting is more appropriate for students who have more severe emotional disabilities or cognitive delays and whose needs cannot be met in the general education setting. Students are generally grouped together by similar educational needs. These classes generally contain a low student-to-staff ratio so that each student is afforded more intensive individual attention (NYC Department of Education 2009).

Home instruction: In cases when a student must be absent for an extended period of time due to her disability, the student is entitled to at least 2 hours daily of instruction at home or in a hospital setting by the state board of education.

Students may move in between these various settings depending on what they need. Parents often fear their child will be "warehoused" in the special education system, but generally once children show gains in their learning or behavior, schools work hard to transition them back into general education settings.

Functional Behavioral Analysis and Positive Behavioral Intervention plans.   When a student who receives IEP services is exhibiting behaviors that disrupt the classroom or the student's learning, the IEP team should perform a **Functional Behavioral Analysis** (FBA) in order to determine the causes of the student's behavior and an effective way to intervene to prevent that behavior from continuing.

The FBA is a structured way in which data are collected to determine what is causing the student's disruptive behavior. Parents and children may be interviewed as well as school staff that interact with the student. The student can also be observed in various settings, such as during recess or lunch, at transitional times, and in the classroom. This assessment should reveal in what context the behavior occurs, factors that influence the behaviors, and how the behavior serves as a function for the student (Jordan 2006). In Kassandra's case, the antecedent may be that she feels helpless and inadequate when she is unable to understand her math work, or perhaps it could be the ending of the school day that triggers these outbursts, because Kassandra knows that she has to return to a home that feels chaotic and unstable.

The findings of the FBA should then influence the **Positive Behavioral Intervention** plan. This plan should be used as a means to develop and reinforce positive behaviors, which should substitute for the disruptive or maladaptive behaviors. This plan can include skill teaching, modeling, making changes to the environment, and providing positive praise and other known effective behavioral modification techniques. FBAs and Positive Behavioral Intervention plans should reflect a student's strength, abilities, and weaknesses and should be tailored to fit the individuality of each student (Jordan 2006).

504 plans.   A 504 plan is an accommodation that can be provided to a student who does not meet eligibility requirements for IEP services when the student has a disability (medical, physical, or mental) that would impair a major life activity but is not severe enough to impair his academic functioning. For instance, an accommodation may be needed for a student who has attention difficulties to be given segmented breaks throughout the class or to be seated closer to the teacher in the room. A child with a medical problem that causes her to be easily fatigued may be given a time in the day in which she is allowed to rest. Typically, documentation is needed from the child's physician in order to apply for 504 accommodations. The school may also require its own evaluation of the child's impairment. Caregivers must request services much as they do for IEP services (National Center for Learning Disabilities 2013).

Day treatment program.　A day treatment program is a more restrictive school-based intervention that often takes place during school day hours and is in many instances located in a hospital setting or community health clinic. This program offers an interdisciplinary approach to providing more intensive interventions than a traditional school setting can offer. Children spend a majority of the day receiving individual, group, and family therapy as well as medication management and activity therapies. Part of the day is spent in educational programming. The model for this program is based on psychosocial and milieu approaches, and cognitive-behavioral treatments are often used.

This programming is more appropriate for students who have received special education services through a traditional school setting but have not been successful in that setting because of the severity of their symptoms. These children are typically struggling with severe psychiatric symptoms, aggression, and/or substance abuse (Thatte et al. 2013). The milieu is highly structured, with small staff-to-child ratio, and staff are highly trained in working with children with special needs. Staff members often include psychiatrists, psychologists, social workers, nurses, activity therapists, and special education teachers. Additional support is provided to families because families will be expected to participate in behavioral programming at home. Programming and services are tailored toward the child's diagnosis and the family's specific needs. The day treatment program is often used as step-down program for children who are transitioning home from inpatient or residential treatment programs or as a preventive measure against having repeated inpatient admissions.

For most day treatment programs, students must have an IEP that reflects an emotional disturbance and indicate that they are not successfully meeting their IEP goals. The child must be engaged with outpatient psychiatric services, and the program is often recommended by the child's treatment team (i.e., therapist, psychologist, psychiatrist) in addition to the school.

Child Welfare, Child Protection, and Other Services for Children and Families

Kassandra's mother is stressed, frustrated, and overwhelmed in her attempts to meet her family's needs and to manage Kassandra's difficult behaviors and symptoms. She admits that, at times, this stress leads her to yell at her children more than she wishes to, and she fears that without help, she might one day hit her children or harm herself.

Kassandra's mother needs help and support, both with parenting and with finding more permanent housing, work or other sources of income, health insurance, social supports, child care, and nutritional assistance.

Although most people think of Child Protective Services (CPS) as only getting involved when children are being frankly abused or endangered, the **child welfare system** actually provides a range of services to ensure safety and strengthen at-risk families before abuse or neglect occurs, to monitor children who are at risk for abuse, and to find permanent homes for children who have been mistreated. The child welfare system is not a single entity but rather a collaboration of many community organizations and private child welfare agencies, overseen by city and state agencies. Child welfare systems are complex, and their specific procedures vary widely by state.

Referrals to child welfare or child protection can be facilitated by hospitals, schools, child welfare agencies, clergy, court/judicial officials, or primary care physicians; by self-referral; or by contacting state or local child welfare department. Services vary from home-based programs to more restrictive or mandatory services, can be voluntary or involuntary, and can take place in various settings such as community-based agencies providing preventative services, in-home family preservation services, foster and therapeutic foster homes, and group placement settings such as group homes, diagnostic evaluation centers, and residential treatment centers (NYC Administration for Children's Services 2014).

Preventative Services

Preventive services. The least restrictive of these services, preventive services work to stabilize at-risk families to prevent abuse or neglect and keep children from entering the child welfare system. Preventive services may include helping families get nutritional assistance or help with rent; respite, which provides short periods of child care to give parents a rest from a difficult child in crisis; trainings and groups for families to learn skills like parenting and anger management; afterschool programs; advocacy; and information and referrals to outpatient clinics. Preventive services workers also help families with vital concrete services such as housing, food, health insurance, employment and financial assistance, mental health care, and substance abuse treatment. Referrals for preventive services are usually made by a CPS worker who has been called to the home to do an investigation, but a family can also go to the preventive services agency directly to request services, or a referral can be made by a pediatrician or another provider. Preventive services are typically voluntary; however, in some cases, preventive services may be mandated by the court after a CPS investigation (NYC Administration for Children's Services 2014).

In-home family preservation services. A more intensive form of preventative services, in-home family preservation services are designed to assist high-risk families involved in the child welfare system with the goal of keeping families together and children safe. Trained professionals work with the identified families by providing extra support, parenting advice, tutoring for children, and help with job and education searches. They work to provide parenting support, improve parenting skills, and promote family functioning while keeping children safe. The goal of the program is to remove the potential for harm and out-of-home placement (NYC Administration for Children's Services 2014).

Preventative services in collaboration with the department of probation. Sometimes parents need help from CPS not because they are at risk for hurting their child or failing to care for him in some way, but because the child is engaging in very dangerous or risky behaviors in defiance of the parent and the parent feels powerless to stop the child. CPS works in collaboration with the family court system to try to help families get these kids back on track, to avoid their getting hurt or arrested. Problems may include running away, truancy, substance misuse or abuse, or refusal to engage in necessary medical and mental health treatment. In these situations, the parent can go to court to request help in supervising and monitoring the child (often called a **person in need of supervision,** or PINS, or a **child in need of supervision,** or CHINS) or, if things are bad enough, a probation officer to help the parent set rules and "police" the child's behavior (NYC Administration for Children's Services 2014).

Foster care placement. In the unfortunate cases when a parent is not able to care for a child, or if there is serious concern for a child's safety while a child protection investigation is being made, children are placed in **foster care.** Foster care can be with a family member (called **kinship foster care**), with a trained foster parent or family, or, if the child has special medical or psychiatric needs, a foster family with extra expertise, training, and support called a **therapeutic foster home.**

Children enter into foster care in one of three ways. The best known pathway into foster care is when a child is judged by CPS to be unsafe at home due to evidence of child abuse and neglect; CPS will bring the case to family court, where the judge will issue an order for the child to be placed into foster care. The other two paths to foster care are placement by a parent's request (so-called **voluntary placement,** as, for example, when the parent is going into the hospital for psychiatric care) and **emergency placement** (as, for example, when a parent dies suddenly and there is no one to care for the child) (NYC Administration for Children's Services 2003).

The CPS team will assess the child's specific needs and assess whether the child can be safely placed in a standard foster home, or whether she needs a therapeutic foster home or a group home or residential placement. **Group homes** and **residential settings** provide children with highly specialized treatment and structure, provided by experienced and trained experts, in a safe, predictable setting. Children and youths served in group home and residential centers today have often been in multiple prior foster homes, experienced significant trauma, or suffered from significant mental health or substance abuse problems. These experiences may lead to problems in school and at home that make it difficult for the child to function in a family or community setting. Since residential settings are considered to be the most restrictive, as they are not located in the community, often residential treatment centers are sought out when a child or youth has failed and exhausted all community supports, services, and interventions (NYS Office of Children and Family Services 2006).

Reporting Abuse and Maltreatment

In the case of Kassandra, mom is stressed and needs support, but there is no evidence of abuse or neglect. In other cases where you suspect abuse or neglect, a report to the State Central Registry is warranted.

The **State Central Register** (SCR), also known as the **"Hotline,"** relays information from the calls to the local CPS for investigation, monitors their prompt response, and identifies if there are prior child abuse or maltreatment reports. It is important to report your concerns as soon as you suspect abuse or maltreatment; even if you are not sure, the SCR staff can help you decide whether there is reason for concern and whether to make a report. Reporting your concerns does not mean you are taking any stand against the family. Your purpose is to assure the safety of the child and the other children in the home. The SCR is available 24 hours, 7 days a week (NYS Office of Children and Family Services 2014). You will be connected to a Child Protective Specialist, who will inform you if CPS has accepted the case and will provide you with a case ID number. If the case is not accepted, you are entitled to speak with a supervisor and take the name of the Child Protective Specialist you spoke with for your records. A CPS worker will contact you to inform you that he or she is currently assigned to the case and may ask for any additional information. Mandated reporters must send the completed 2221A to the field office in the borough where the subjects of the report reside within 48 hours of making a report to the SCR.

Services for Children
With Developmental Disabilities

While Kassandra does not have a formal diagnosis of autism spectrum disorder, she does show many symptoms that are suggestive of autism, including difficulties in managing transitions, self-soothing behaviors such as rocking, and self-injurious behaviors such as biting during meltdowns. If, after a full assessment, Kassandra is found to have autism spectrum disorder or another developmental disability, she will benefit from special services targeted to her cognitive and developmental level.

Although children with autism, developmental disabilities, and intellectual disabilities are often treated in the mental health system, there is actually a wholly separate network of programs dedicated to helping children with intellectual and developmental disabilities (I/DD). Some services are funded through the county or state, but most are funded by the federal government through Medicaid.

Getting Connected

Getting connected to services for children with I/DD can be more complicated than simply scheduling an intake at a clinic; in most states, a child must be determined to be eligible by the state office that administers such programs (in New York, it is called the Office for People With Developmental Disabilities, or OPWDD; www.opwdd.ny.gov). Eligibility criteria differ from state to state, but in New York State the requirement is that the individual has a diagnosed developmental disability that started before the age of 22 and is expected to continue indefinitely or permanently and that causes a substantial handicap to the person's functioning.

Qualifying conditions include autism, intellectual disability, cerebral palsy, epilepsy, familial dysautonomia, and neurological impairment (i.e., injury, malformation, or disease involving the central nervous system). Eligibility status can be reviewed from infancy throughout a person's life. It is important to be aware, however, that the older a person is at eligibility determination, the harder it may be to document proof of disability onset before age 22. The process of applying or determining eligibility is different in every state as well; in New York State, OPWDD has a single point of access similar to that in the mental health system, known as the "Front Door."

Types of Services for Children
With Developmental Disabilities

Having a family member with a developmental disability can be overwhelming at times. Many services are available, but families often need assistance in navigating the system for access to services and advocating on behalf of their loved one.

Services and supports that states offer to families with children with I/DD include respite services; financial services such as cash subsidies and vouchers; in-home supports such as personal assistance or homemaker services; assistive technology and environmental modification; adaptive medical equipment; health and professional services; therapies; family counseling; family training; parent support groups; transportation; recreation activities; specialized clothing; and dietary services.

Case management and service coordination.   Like the case managers in the mental health system, case managers and service coordinators in the I/DD system help get the child connected with the right services, and help parents manage the various appointments and stay connected to care.

Clinic services.   Although many children with I/DD are treated in the mental health system, specialized clinics run by the I/DD system can offer many more services than do mental health clinics. These services include primary medical, dental, and social work supports as well as **occupational therapy, physical therapy,** psychology, psychiatry, **rehabilitation counseling, speech and language therapy, audiological testing,** and **social skills training** to help a child learn to function as successfully and independently as possible.

Intensive behavioral therapies.   Behavioral interventions are key for individuals with autism spectrum disorder and other developmental disabilities, and children who are eligible through the I/DD system can access **intensive home-based behavioral treatments,** including FBA; specialized behavioral therapies such as **Applied Behavior Analysis**; and behavior management plans, implementation and monitoring of behavioral interventions, and training in the behavior management plan. All of these interventions should be available to children with autism spectrum disorder or other developmental disabilities through the I/DD system and/or through the board of education.

Services for Families and Caregivers

Caring for a child with an intellectual or developmental disability can be very difficult and stressful for families, so the I/DD service system offers additional supports for patients and families, including respite, recreation, counseling, and advocacy.

Respite programs (short-term caregiver relief). Respite programs provide short-term relief to parents and caregivers who are responsible for the primary care and support of individuals with disabilities. Services are provided by the hour and are available during the day, over the weekend, or overnight. Respite can occur in a person's home or at an approved site, such as a freestanding respite center. Respite gives a parent or caregiver an emotional break and an opportunity to attend appointments, get groceries, or do other things that they cannot do while accompanied by their I/DD child.

Recreational programs. Many children with I/DD do not do well in typical afterschool or sports programs, so special recreational programs exist to let them have social and leisure activities—after school, on weekends, or at summer camp—in a supported setting.

Counseling, training, and supports. Counseling, training, and educational activities and supports may be available for parents, siblings, and caregivers, as well as for individuals with developmental disabilities. These services may be helpful for individuals and families who are looking to gain insight, resolve problems, develop alternative approaches to services, and address other issues of concern.

Advocacy. Advocacy may include information and referral services, outreach, parent networking, and service assistance for individuals and their families. It is possible to make connections with diagnostic, residential, rehabilitative, educational, vocational, medical, and recreational services, and with other programs such as Medicaid and Supplemental Security Income.

Home and Community-Based Services Waiver

As discussed earlier in this chapter, a HCBS or "waiver" provides intensive home-based services for children and adolescents with severe difficulties or needs. Just as the mental health system offers this service for children with severe mental health needs, waiver services are available to children with I/DD through the I/DD system.

Foster Care for Children With Special Needs

When children with I/DD need foster care, they are placed with families who have received special training and certification by the I/DD system. They also receive additional supports, such as a family care coordinator, family care providers, Medicaid service coordinators, and a nursing team that provides medical care and intervention.

Residential Placement and Residential Schools for Children With Autism Spectrum Disorder

Some children with autism require such a high level of caretaking and support that they cannot be safely cared for in a family home (either their own or a specialized foster home). It can be a difficult and painful decision for a family to take the step of placing their child in care, and these decisions are never made lightly. The therapists, case manager, and school staff should help the family to make this decision and to find the right placement for the child. Some children are placed for a year or two for intensive therapy, while others require that intensive level of support far into adulthood (NYC Administration for Children's Services 2003).

Connecting Kids to the Right Resources

As demonstrated throughout this chapter, there is a wide range of resources available to kids and families, and a trip to the ER is not required to access them. It is crucial that you become familiar with the various resources that are available within the community to properly refer children and families to the services that best fit the child's mental health issues. Clinicians should learn the nuances of how the referral process works for each type of intervention, as this may vary from state to state and community to community. It can be helpful to meet and collaborate with administrators and clinicians from community-based agencies in order to have a solid understanding of the services they offer and of how to make connections for the children and families you work with. Knowledge of community-based services can also better inform your evaluation and can help you to collaborate with families and caregivers to help pick the best interventions possible.

In some communities there are ample resources, whereas in other communities services may be lacking. You can be a crucial advocate for the children and families with which you work, to push politicians and policymakers to invest in therapeutic resources and develop services in your community.

References

Jordan J: Functional Behavioral Assessment and positive interventions: what parents need to know (Pacer Center Action Information Sheet). Minneapolis, MN, Pacer Center, 2006. Available at: http://www.pacer.org/parent/php/php-c79.pdf. Accessed May 5, 2014.

Massachusetts General Hospital, School Psychiatry Program and MADI Resource Center: School-based interventions: before you begin, 2010. Available at: http://www2.massgeneral.org/schoolpsychiatry/interventions_begin.asp. Accessed September 11, 2013.

National Center for Learning Disabilities: Section 504 and IDEA comparison chart. Available at: http://www.ncld.org/disability-advocacy/learn-ld-laws/adaaa-section-504/section-504-idea-comparison-chart. Accessed October 15, 2013.

NYC Administration for Children's Services: Parent Handbook: A Guide for Parents With Children in Foster Care, February 2003. Available at: http://www.nycpartnersforfamilies.org/wp-content/uploads/2010/03/ACS-Parent-Handbook.pdf. Accessed October 11, 2013.

NYC Administration for Children's Services: Support for families, 2014. Available at:http://www.nyc.gov/html/acs/html/support_families/support_families.shtml. Accessed May 13, 2014.

NYC Department of Education: Community and high school superintendents: district and borough family advocates. Available at: http://schools.nyc.gov/AboutUs/schools/superintendents/DFAcontact.htm. Accessed September 2, 2013.

NYC Department of Education, Office of Special Education Initiatives: Special Education Services as Part of a Unified Service Delivery System, 2009. Available at: http://schools.nyc.gov/NR/rdonlyres/C7A58626-6637-42E7-AD00-70440820661D/0/ContinuumofServices.pdf. Accessed October 15, 2013.

NYC Department of Health and Mental Hygiene: Community mental health supports and services, 2012a. Available at: http://www.nyc.gov/html/doh/html/mental/child-services-community.shtml. Accessed May 13, 2014.

NYC Department of Health and Mental Hygiene: Community residential services, 2012b. Available at: http://www.nyc.gov/html/doh/html/mental/child-services-residential.shtml. Accessed September 14, 2013.

NYC Department of Health and Mental Hygiene: Mobile crisis team, 2012c. Available at: http://www.nyc.gov/html/doh/html/mental/mobile-crisis.shtml. Accessed May 13, 2014.

NYC Department of Health and Mental Hygiene: Home based crisis intervention, 2013. Available at: http://www.nyc.gov/html/doh/html/mental/child-services-crisis.shtml. Accessed May 13, 2014.

NYC Department of Youth and Community Development: Case management standards toolkit. [2011] Available at: http://www.nyc.gov/html/dycd/downloads/pdf/NYC_DYCD_Case_Management_Toolkit-2011.pdf. Accessed May 13, 2014.

NYS Office of Children and Family Services: Child Protective Services. Available at: http://www.ocfs.state.ny.us/main/cps. Accessed May 1, 2014.

NYS Office of Children and Family Services: Residential Care in New York State: 2006 and Beyond, December 18, 2006. Available at: http://ocfs.ny.gov/main/policies/external/OCFS_2006/INFs/06-OCFS-INF-09%20Residential%20Care%20in%20New%20York%20State%20-%202006%20and%20Beyond.pdf. Accessed October 11, 2013.

Price-Ellingstad D, Reynolds J, Ringer L, et al: A Guide to the Individualized Education Program. July 2000. Available at: http://www2.ed.gov/parents/needs/speced/iepguide/index.html. Accessed August 23, 2013.

Thatte S, Makinen J, Nguyen H, et al: Partial hospitalization for youth with psychiatric disorders: treatment outcomes and 3-month follow-up. J Nerv Ment Dis 201(5):429–434, 2013

U.S. Public Health Service: Report of the Surgeon General's Conference on Children's Mental Health: A National Action Agenda. Washington, DC, Department of Health and Human Services, 2000. Available at: http://www.ncbi.nlm.nih.gov/books/NBK44233. Accessed May 1, 2014.

CHAPTER 11

Models of Emergency Psychiatric Care for Children and Adolescents

Moving From Triage to Meaningful Engagement in Mental Health Treatment

Jennifer F. Havens, M.D.
Mollie C. Marr, B.F.A.

The dramatic increase in visits to emergency rooms (ERs) by children and adolescents in psychiatric crisis that began in the 1990s has persisted into the twenty-first century, with the latest estimates of pediatric ER visits for behavioral health issues ranging from 2% to 5% of all visits (Grover and Lee 2013; Pittsenbarger and Mannix 2011; Sills and Bland 2002). As other parts of the mental health care system constrict (Cummings et al. 2013; Geller and Biebel 2006; New Freedom Commission on Mental Health 2004), the emergency department (ED) increasingly serves as the mental health safety net. Unfortunately, the emergency care system has been slow to evolve to meet the needs of these young patients, who present significant burdens to most EDs, with longer stays and increased need for admission/transfer than other young patients (Case et al. 2011; Dolan and Fein 2011; Grover and Lee 2013; Grupp-Phelan et al. 2009; Santiago et al. 2006; Waseem et al. 2011).

Across the country, young patients are generally managed in either medical EDs or adult psychiatry settings. Both of these settings commonly lack round-the-clock access to child and adolescent psychiatric clinicians; young patients in psychiatric crisis are evaluated and managed by clinical staff without specific expertise in child and adolescent assessment and treatment planning, particularly on nights and weekends. In addition, medical or pediatric EDs lack the physical facilities to safely manage psychiatric patients, including a holding space free of objects that can be used when there is risk of self-harm and locked facilities (to prevent elopement of high-risk patients). Managing young patients in adult psychiatric settings (which have more appropriate physical space than do medical settings) presents another set of problems, including the often traumatizing nature of these settings as well as the lack of child and adolescent expertise.

Young patients present to emergency settings in varying degrees of acuity. Some of these presentations relate to difficulties accessing routine services and reflect the lack of capacity in the child outpatient system and, in particular, access to child psychiatrists. Because emergency settings generally lack any capacity to provide ongoing engagement and treatment services, these patients are poorly served by attempts to use the ER to enter the mental health system. As there is generally little to no capacity to provide care to acutely ill children and adolescents in the outpatient clinic system, the only option for patients at higher levels of acuity is admission to inpatient units. Across the United States between 30% and 40% of pediatric psychiatric emergency presentations result in inpatient admission (Case et al. 2011; Mahajan et al. 2009; Pottick et al. 1995; Sills and Bland 2002). With the steady decline in access to inpatient child and adolescent psychiatry beds (Geller and Biebel 2006; New Freedom Commission on Mental Health 2004), the system is often backlogged and young people are boarded in EDs or on pediatric units awaiting inpatient admission (Case et al. 2011; Wharff et al. 2011).

The problems underlying the deficiencies in the psychiatric emergency response capacity are complex and multifactorial. First, the pressures on EDs to manage psychiatric patients have increased for all age groups (Grupp-Phelan et al. 2009; Larkin et al. 2005; Sills and Bland 2002). This increasing reliance on EDs reflects both limitations in access to routine and preventive mental health care secondary to insurance and reimbursement issues and the ongoing trend toward reduction in both numbers of public and private inpatient beds and length of stay of inpatient psychiatric admissions (Cummings et al. 2013; New Freedom Commission on Mental Health 2004; Pottick et al. 2001; Thomas 2003). Second, the common model of psychiatry consultation to EDs is generally associated with little to no direct reimbursement, particularly in those settings serving indigent populations. This lack of direct reimbursement limits the resources available to support psychiatric staffing. Third, workforce issues in child and adolescent psychiatry make the problem particularly severe for young patients; immediate access to clinical staff with child and adolescent psychiatric expertise is a huge challenge in the best of circumstances and is generally limited to large academic medical centers with significant training programs. This combination of lack of financial support for mental health service delivery and workforce limitations is the foundation of the current child psychiatric emergency care system, which does not meet the needs of the growing numbers of young people accessing EDs for urgent or emergent mental health problems.

Across the country, providers and systems struggling with these issues have developed a number of emerging models to improve care for young people in psychiatric crisis. These models include community-based programs with intensive in-home supports; hospital-based clinic models that provide rapid access to outpatient services; ED-based programs that provide enhanced evaluation and referral support; and dedicated child and adolescent psychiatric emergency programs that provide brief stabilization and immediate follow-up treatment.

Despite the variety of organizational structures, the models share essential common features. First, they provide immediate access to clinical staff with expertise in the management of child and adolescent psychiatric crisis. Second, they support children and families through the crisis period and provide facilitated linkage to ongoing services. Third, they are supported by revenue streams that allow the delivery of flexible services that meet the needs of the child and family, often in the home. Many of these models have been shown to be effective and to reduce rates of hospital admission (Janssens et al. 2013; Pumariega and Winters 2003; Shepperd et al. 2009). Since 30%–40% of current presentations of youths in psychiatric emergency result in inpatient admission, these models have the potential to reduce inpatient utilization and facilitate access to ongoing mental health treatment. These programs are described in detail in the following sections.

Community-Based Models

Two well-established evidence-based models of intensive community-based care have been adapted to serve children in psychiatric emergencies. The

Homebuilders model, originally designed to support family preservation in child welfare populations (Forsythe 1992; Kinney et al. 1977), has been successfully utilized to prevent psychiatric admissions in youths (Evans et al. 1997, 2003). The New York State Office of Mental Health has invested in the **home-based crisis intervention** model and supports a network of such programs in New York City. This model provides short-term in-home services (6–12 weeks) and linkage to outpatient services to children and adolescents who have been identified as being at risk for psychiatric hospitalization. This model successfully diverts over 90% of young people from psychiatric admission and has been found to successfully manage patients at the same level of acuity as those admitted to inpatient services (Lyons 2004).

The second model, **multisystemic therapy** (MST), has been adapted to serve youths at risk of psychiatric hospitalization and has also been shown to be effective in safely managing these youths (Henggeler et al. 1999). Similar to the Homebuilders model, this model provides home-based services, but with a variable intensity and longer length of treatment (average of 4 months) based on the needs of the family. MST combines family, behavioral, and psychosocial interventions to assist families in identifying and using available resources and family strengths to enact change. For children in psychiatric crisis, MST was adapted to focus on the development of comprehensive crisis plans, and the treatment team was expanded to include child and adolescent psychiatrists (Henggeler et al. 1999, 2003). This model prevented hospitalization for 57% of patients enrolled in a randomized controlled study of MST versus hospitalization following a psychiatric crisis (Schoenwald et al. 2000) and reduced suicide attempts in youths referred for hospitalization for suicidal ideation/suicide attempt or threats of harm to self or others (Huey et al. 2004).

An additional community-based model, with a growing evidence base, is **mobile crisis services.** Mobile crisis teams go to the site of crisis (home, school, community) and provide onsite evaluation to determine if the child needs a higher level of care, short-term wraparound services, and referral and linkage to outpatient services. Mobile crisis teams are also used to contact high-risk patients following an ED visit or hospitalization either to encourage linkage or to look into failure to attend scheduled appointments (Currier et al. 2010). The mobile crisis team in Milwaukee, Wisconsin, is able to facilitate transfer to a local inpatient program or access to crisis respite beds and has been shown to decrease inpatient admissions (Pumariega and Winters 2003). A similar program in New York reduced ED visits and prevented out-of-home placements (Shulman and Athey 1993). Although there is a growing literature supporting the use of mobile crisis teams to reduce hospitalizations in adults, data specific to children and adolescents remain limited.

One significant barrier to the broader implementation of community-based models is the requirement for ongoing external funding to support program costs. Despite the clear cost savings from hospital diversions, these types of services are generally not covered by insurance providers. Strategic collaboration with insurers (both commercial and public) is essential to the successful dissemination of these program models.

Hospital-Based Models

Hospital-based models include specialized crisis intervention teams that provide hospital-based services, either on a walk-in basis or as an immediate disposition from the ER. These programs are generally co-located with other clinic services but provide immediate access to clinical teams with expertise in crisis intervention (Blumberg 2002). This model has the most applicability to existing clinic services and represents an evolution in outpatient care to include an acute care capability. Recently, some clinics have implemented adaptations of routine outpatient care that allow **rapid access to specialized teams providing intensive management of patients in crisis,** allowing for discharge from EDs of patients who can be managed in outpatient settings. This model generally works best in an academic setting with trainees, who increase access to child psychiatry services. One innovative model developed at Maimonides Medical Center in Brooklyn, New York, involves **active linkage to local public schools** with the capacity for urgent evaluations of students every day of the work week. This model allows schools to send students for walk-in outpatient evaluation with facilitated communication to the clinic crisis providers, preventing some school referrals to the emergency setting.

Emergency Department–Based Models

There are three main approaches addressed by ED-based models: conducting enhanced evaluation and referral, providing therapeutic interventions within the ED during the initial visit, and supporting dedicated psychiatric staff within the ED (child guidance model). These models expand existing ED services and move beyond the traditional psychiatric consult model.

The **enhanced evaluation and referral** model includes facilitated referral to outpatient services by ED staff, review of expectations and verbal contracting about safety, crisis phone support, and reminder phone calls to help families connect with outpatient services (Janssens et al. 2013; Newton et al. 2010). The **therapeutic intervention** model, like the enhanced evaluation and referral model, has been evaluated with high-risk patients typically presenting with suicidal ideation or self-inflicted injury. Several family-based crisis interventions have been evaluated. These interventions combine brief family systems therapy, cognitive-behavioral therapy, or a combination of therapeutic techniques to help the child and parents reframe the crisis, identify how to establish and maintain safety, improve communication, and address attitudes about pursuing mental health care (Rotheram-Borus et al. 2000; Wharff et al. 2012). The Rotheram-Borus et al. (2000) study included linkage calls to provide support and increase compliance with outpatient follow-up appointments. Both the Rotheram-Borus et al. study and the Wharff et al. study found improved linkage and compliance with outpatient services following the ED-based interventions (Rotheram-Borus et al. 2000; Wharff et al. 2012).

In the **child guidance** model (Mahajan et al. 2007), a team comprising a psychiatric social worker and a child psychiatrist evaluates all children and adolescents presenting with psychiatric complaints. The psychiatric social worker is available in the ED 24 hours a day and is able to provide psychiatric assessment and comprehensive disposition planning. Mahajan et al. (2007) found that the presence of the child guidance team reduced the length of stay in the ED as well as costs. Similar interventions involving pediatric psychiatric teams providing evaluation and disposition planning in the ED led to a reduction in inpatient admissions and return ED visits (Hamm et al. 2010).

Specialty Psychiatric Emergency Programs

Specialized, dedicated child and adolescent psychiatric emergency programs with brief stabilization facilities are feasible in higher-volume settings (e.g., 2,000 emergency psychiatric visits per year) but require considerable capital investment and institutional commitment to develop and implement, because they are expensive to build and operate and require a critical mass of child psychiatry staffing. The first dedicated Children's Comprehensive Psychiatric Emergency Program (C-CPEP) in New York State (at New York Presbyterian Hospital) reduced inpatient psychiatric admissions in Northern Manhattan from 35% to under 10%, but was closed when inadequate volume and reimbursement did not support program costs. The second dedicated C-CPEP in New York State (at Bellevue Hospital Center) serves both Bellevue Hospital and several other public hospitals in the

New York City Health and Hospitals Corporation that lack child and adolescent inpatient services. The C-CPEP includes six extended observation beds staffed 24 hours a day/7 days a week with child psychiatry, nursing, and social work. The service also provides Interim Crisis Clinic services, which follow patients discharged from the C-CPEP for up to five visits. This combination of immediate access to outpatient follow-up and brief stabilization prevents longer admissions except when necessary; only 20% of children and adolescents evaluated in Bellevue C-CPEP are admitted to inpatient psychiatry units. A similar specialized program was opened at the Institute of Living in Hartford, Connecticut (the CARES Unit), in 2009, in response to the dramatic increase in young people in psychiatric crisis in medical EDs in that state. Another brief stabilization unit has been opened in Geneva, Switzerland, at the Children's Hospital of University Hospitals of Geneva.

Moving Forward

There is an array of service models that address the limitations of the existing service system, and these models can be tailored to sites with varying volume. Although there is little systematic research guiding the selection of these models (Hamm et al. 2010; Janssens et al. 2013; Lamb 2009; Shepperd et al. 2009), there is clear preliminary evidence that enhancing the service system's ability to serve young people and families in crisis has the potential to reduce inpatient utilization and to more effectively engage patients in ongoing mental health treatment.

Extensive advocacy is necessary on a national level to force the development of standards of care and ensure adequate reimbursement for pediatric psychiatric emergency care. Following the path of emergency medicine and accrediting and designating centers of child and adolescent psychiatric emergency care could improve the accessibility of quality care, facilitate patient transfer and linkage, and create an infrastructure for innovation, research, and training. The designation process developed by the Illinois Emergency Medical Services for Children program led to the development of statewide standards and protocols for provision of emergency medical care to children and engaged providers across service systems, including emergency medical services, schools, rehabilitation centers, poison control centers, and hospitals (Lyons 2014). The program has been able to leverage the partnerships formed as part of the designation process to advance disaster preparedness, develop a surveillance system, implement and evaluate system-wide quality improvement projects, and address workforce, equipment, and space shortages. The designation process is based on the ability of hospitals to provide optimal pediatric care and encompasses three levels of pediatric capabilities. Hospitals, especially those centers unable to provide specialized pediatric care, must have transfer guidelines in place. The system facilitates medically necessary pediatric transfers both through the requirement of current policies and interagency agreements and by maintaining up-to-date information on the location and availability of transportation teams, specialized centers of care, and pediatric beds. Accrediting and designating centers of child and adolescent psychiatric emergency care is an important next step in ensuring access to high-quality care and providing the infrastructure to evaluate and improve the existing service system and support the development of new models of care.

References

Blumberg SH: Crisis intervention program: an alternative to inpatient psychiatric treatment for children. Ment Health Serv Res 4(1):1–6, 2002

Case SD, Case BG, Olfson M, et al: Length of stay of pediatric mental health emergency department visits in the United States. J Am Acad Child Adolesc Psychiatry 50:1110–1119, 2011

Cummings JR, Wen H, Druss BG: Improving access to mental health services for youth in the United States. JAMA 309(6):553–554, 2013

Currier GW, Fisher SG, Caine ED: Mobile crisis team intervention to enhance linkage of discharged suicidal emergency department patients to outpatient psychiatric services: a randomized controlled trial. Acad Emerg Med 17(1):36–43, 2010

Dolan MA, Fein JA: Pediatric and adolescent mental health emergencies in the emergency medical services system. Pediatrics 127(5):e1356–e1366, 2011

Evans ME, Boothroyd RA, Armstrong MI: Development and implementation of an experimental study of the effectiveness of intensive in-home crisis services for children and their families. Journal of Emotional and Behavioral Disorders 5(2):93–105, 1997

Evans ME, Boothroyd RA, Armstrong MI, et al: An experimental study of the effectiveness of intensive in-home crisis services for children and their families program outcomes. Journal of Emotional and Behavioral Disorders 11(2):92–102, 2003

Forsythe P: Homebuilders and family preservation. Children and Youth Services Review 14(1):37–47, 1992

Geller JL, Biebel K: The premature demise of public child and adolescent inpatient psychiatric beds. Psychiatr Q 77(3):251–271, 2006

Grover P, Lee T: Dedicated pediatric behavioral health unit: serving the unique and individual needs of children in behavioral health crisis. Pediatr Emerg Care 29(2):200–202, 2013

Grupp-Phelan J, Mahajan P, Foltin GL, et al: Referral and resource use patterns for psychiatric-related visits to pediatric emergency departments. Pediatr Emerg Care 25(4):217–220, 2009

Hamm MP, Osmond M, Curran J, et al: A systematic review of crisis interventions used in the emergency department: recommendations for pediatric care and research. Pediatr Emerg Care 26(12):952–962, 2010

Henggeler SW, Rowland MD, Randall J, et al: Home-based multisystemic therapy as an alternative to the hospitalization of youths in psychiatric crisis: clinical outcomes. J Am Acad Child Adolesc Psychiatry 38(11):1331–1339, 1999

Henggeler SW, Rowland MD, Halliday-Boykins CA, et al: One-year follow-up of multisystemic therapy as an alternative to the hospitalization of youths in psychiatric crisis. J Am Acad Child Adolesc Psychiatry 42(5):543–551, 2003

Huey SJ, Henggeler SW, Rowland MD, et al: Multisystemic therapy effects on attempted suicide by youths presenting psychiatric emergencies. J Am Acad Child Adolesc Psychiatry 43(2):183–190, 2004

Janssens A, Hayen S, Walraven V, et al: Emergency psychiatric care for children and adolescents: a literature review. Pediatr Emerg Care 29(9):1041–1050, 2013

Kinney JM, Madsen B, Fleming T, Haapala DA: Homebuilders: keeping families together. J Consult Clin Psychol 45(4):667–673, 1977

Lamb CE: Alternatives to admission for children and adolescents: providing intensive mental healthcare services at home and in communities: what works? Curr Opin Psychiatry 22(4):345–350, 2009

Larkin GL, Claassen CA, Emond JA, et al: Trends in US emergency department visits for mental health conditions, 1992 to 2001. Psychiatr Serv 56(6):671–677, 2005

Lyons E: Illinois Emergency Medical Services for Children, facility recognition, March 19, 2014. Available at: http://www.luhs.org/depts/emsc/facility.htm. Accessed April 14, 2014.

Lyons JS: Redressing the Emperor: Improving Our Children's Public Mental Health System. Westport, CT, Praeger, 2004

Mahajan P, Thomas R, Rosenberg DR, et al: Evaluation of a child guidance model for visits for mental disorders to an inner-city pediatric emergency department. Pediatr Emerg Care 23(4):212–217, 2007

Mahajan P, Alpern ER, Grupp-Phelan J, et al: Epidemiology of psychiatric-related visits to emergency departments in a multicenter collaborative research pediatric network. Pediatr Emerg Care 25(11):715–720, 2009

New Freedom Commission on Mental Health, Subcommittee on Acute Care: background paper (DHHS Publ No SMA-04-3876). Rockville, MD, June 2004

Newton AS, Hamm MP, Bethell J, et al: Pediatric suicide-related presentations: a systematic review of mental health care in the emergency department. Ann Emerg Med 56(6):649–659, 2010

Pittsenbarger Z, Mannix R: Disproportionately increasing psychiatric visits to the pediatric emergency department among the underinsured. Abstract presented at the annual meeting of the American Academy of Pediatrics, Boston, MA, October 2011

Pottick K, Hansell S, Gutterman E, White HR: Factors associated with inpatient and outpatient treatment for children and adolescents with serious mental illness. J Am Acad Child Adolesc Psychiatry 34(4):425–433, 1995

Pottick KJ, Barber CC, Hansell S, Coyne L: Changing patterns of inpatient care for children and adolescents at the Menninger Clinic, 1988–1994. J Consult Clin Psychol 69(3):573–577, 2001

Pumariega AJ, Winters NC: Trends and shifting ecologies, Part II. Child Adolesc Psychiatr Clinics N Am 12(4):779–793, 2003

Rotheram-Borus MJ, Piacentini J, Cantwell C, et al: The 18-month impact of an emergency room intervention for adolescent female suicide attempters. J Consult Clin Psychol 68(6):1081–1093, 2000

Santiago L, Tunik M, Foltin G, Mojica M: Children requiring psychiatric consultation in the pediatric emergency department: epidemiology, resource utilization, and complications. Pediatr Emerg Care 22(2):85–89, 2006

Schoenwald SK, Ward DM, Henggeler SW, Rowland MD: Multisystemic therapy versus hospitalization for crisis stabilization of youth: placement outcomes 4 months postreferral. Ment Health Serv Res 2(1):3–12, 2000

Shepperd S, Doll H, Gowers S, et al: Alternatives to inpatient mental health care for children and young people. Cochrane Database Syst Rev CD006410, April 15, 2009

Shulman DA, Athey M: Youth emergency services: total community effort, a multisystem approach. Child Welfare: Journal of Policy, Practice, and Program 72(2):171–179, 1993

Sills MR, Bland SD: Summary statistics for pediatric psychiatric visits to US emergency departments, 1993–1999. Pediatrics 110(4):e40-e40, 2002

Thomas LE: Trends and shifting ecologies, Part I. Child Adolesc Psychiatr Clin N Am 12(4):599–611, 2003

Waseem M, Prasankumar R, Pagan K, Leber M: A retrospective look at length of stay for pediatric psychiatric patients in an urban emergency department. Pediatr Emerg Care 27(3):170–173, 2011

Wharff EA, Ginnis KB, Ross AM, Blood EA: Predictors of psychiatric boarding in the pediatric emergency department: implications for emergency care. Pediatr Emerg Care 27(6):483–489, 2011

Wharff EA, Ginnis KM, Ross AM: Family-based crisis intervention with suicidal adolescents in the emergency room: a pilot study. Soc Work 57(2):133–143, 2012

Index

Page numbers printed in **boldface** *refer to tables or figures.*